# The Patient Comes FIRST

# The Patient Comes FIRST

## A Nurse Speaks Out

**NANCY FOX**

Illustrations by Ulf G. Hansell
Edited by Harold R. Gillespie, Jr.

PROMETHEUS BOOKS
Buffalo, New York

Published 1988 by
Prometheus Books
700 E. Amherst Street, Buffalo, New York 14215
Printed in the United States of America

Copyright © 1988 by Nancy Fox

First published in 1985 by Geriatric Press, Inc., Bend, Oregon.

All rights reserved. No part of this publication may be reproduced, stored in a retrieval system, or transmitted, in any form or by any means, electronic, mechanical, photocopying, recording or otherwise, without the prior permission of the publisher.

ISBN 0-87975-479-6
Library of Congress Catalog Card Number: 88-61282

# TABLE OF CONTENTS

### PART ONE: *HOSPITALS*
### "The Quality of Mercy?"

CHAPTER
1. Haven or Horror-Chamber? Your Hospital ICU ............... 1
2. Call to Arms:
   Just *What* Do We Want for Our Mentally Ill? ............... 11
3. Visible vs. Invisible Nursing: Never Show Emotion? ........ 21

### PART TWO: *NURSING HOMES*
### A Generation in Jeopardy?

4. Is This "Senility" Necessary? Wring out the Old! ............ 29
5. Murder by Nutrition: It Takes a Cast-Iron Stomach! ......... 39
6. Who *Me?* A Nursing Home Resident? ........................ 47
7. Personal Possessions: Trash or Treasure? ..................... 59
8. The Shush-up of Mrs. Park: Aftermath of Stroke ............. 65
9. Sexuality at *Any* Age: Part of Being Human ................. 79

### PART THREE: *RETIREMENT*
### Blueprint for Oblivion?

10. Mothers'/Fathers' Day - In China? Unheard Of! ............. 93
11. Those Magazine Ads: You Did a Doubletake? ............... 103
12. Don't Rush the Rocking Chair! ............................... 109

### PART FOUR: *A SOCIETAL ISSUE -*
### . . . of the "stickiest" kind

13. *Euthan* . . . or *Dysthan-asia?*
    Pretend It's *You!* ............................................. 121

### EPILOGUE

### TO MAKE MEANINGFUL THEIR DAYS:
### Is Living Longer *Really* Living Better?

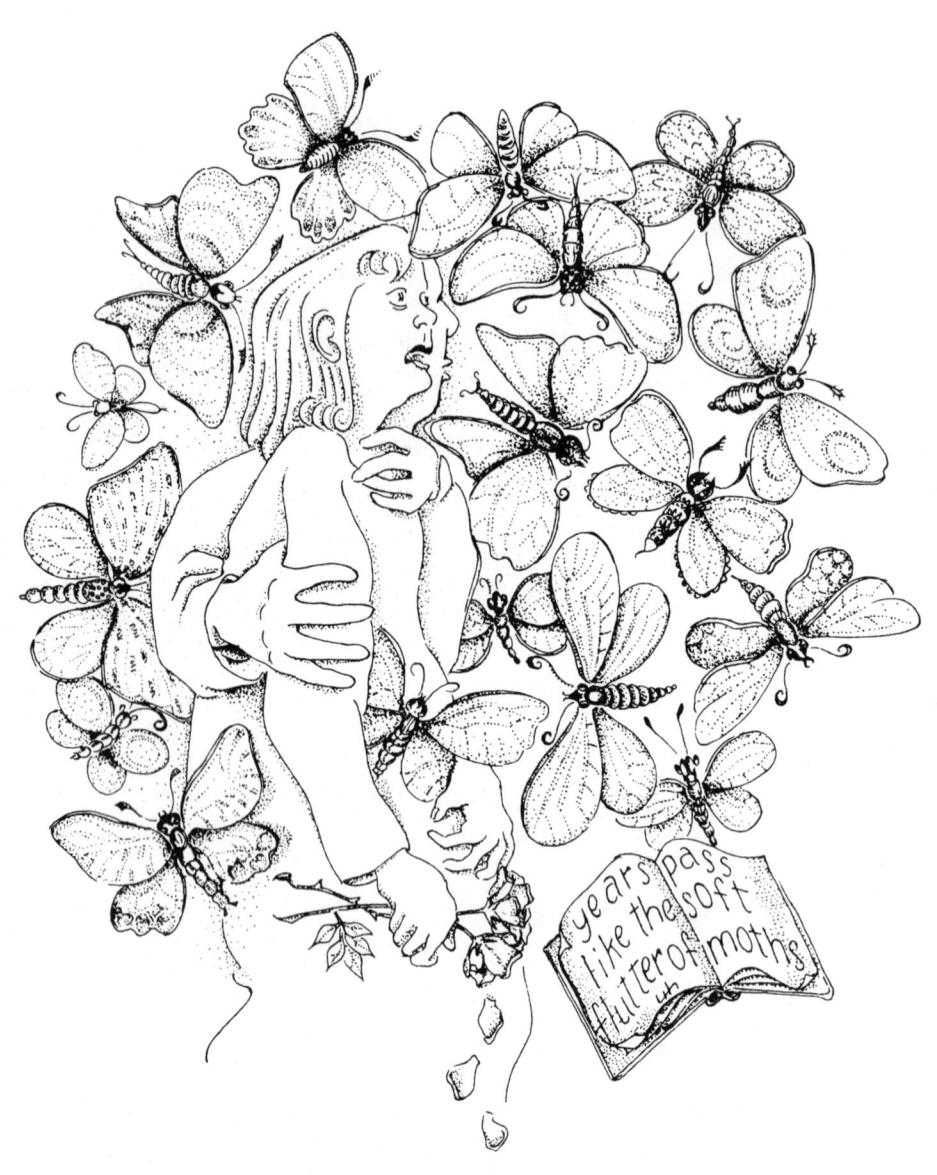

# PREFACE

This book is unconventional. Each chapter, unrelated to the next, dwells on a specific concern in today's health care field. You might view this work as an anthology in which a nurse confronts issues both sociologically and from a personal experience vantage point.

For good reason, chapters six and ten shift in tone from the "sticky" issue theme, partly as relief for the reader, partly because these two essays serve as models for the entire health care industry. They describe programs whose simple philosophy: "THE PATIENT COMES FIRST" is put to actual practice.

Following her own nationwide survey of health care institutions, the author concludes that despite serious inequities, there exist *some* "good" facilities. A handful. However, by focusing on deep-seated, unresolved, issues, the reader may gain impetus to act, to speak up, to help balance our lopsided scale of priorities. Now is not too soon. We dare wait no longer. The years pass for each of us, "like the soft flutter of moths." And then, what for ourselves will *we* want? What will *we* expect in the way of healthcare?

Referring to chapter one, Norman Cousins, author of *Anatomy of an Illness*, observes: "You have touched upon some valid points." Indeed, throughout the book, valid points cry out to gain, not just our awareness, but our efforts to induce drastic changes; to humanize these places whose "cures" often succeed visibly but which so rarely speak to the inner needs of human beings in distress.

Not until as a nation we adopt that simple slogan: "THE PATIENT COMES FIRST" can we square our shoulders and, in all honesty, tell the world: "We've got it made! In the field of healthcare, America is the greatest!"

NOTE: To spare the reader that repetitious he/she and him/her syndrome, the author decided to toss a coin. Heads, *he* — tails, *she*. Heads won!

All names of persons or places are fictitious, except where otherwise indicated.

# PART ONE: *HOSPITALS*
## "The Quality of Mercy?"

*Tremendous, our U.S. technology!*
*But when is it too much?*

## CHAPTER ONE

# HAVEN FOR HELP OR HORROR-CHAMBER?
## Your Hospital ICU

## Haven for Help or Horror-Chamber?
## Your Hospital ICU

I had heard about the ICU, that secretive Intensive Care Unit, that sealed-off inner-sanctum where under time-bomb pressure split-second life-death decisions are made. Years ago, as a student nurse I had toured such a place. And I'd read about that "Forbidden City," where only next-of-kin may visit; about the patients in there, victims of stroke, shock, hemorrhage, accidents, heart-attacks, aneurysm, fracture and suicide-murder attempts.

Yes, I knew about this wonderland of science and technology containing a million dollars worth of equipment that might produce medical miracles — a maze of machines which determine the state of, the fate of struggling or blanked-out bodies on high-rise beds. And I'd heard of those physicians — emperors reigning over their subjects, the medical support staff.

These were simply images in my mind — images, that is, until the day when the medics wheeled my spouse into an ICU. The vague images then came into focus. But not all at once. At that point I was too distraught. But as the hours passed I began to sort out impressions — the sights, sounds smells of an ICU. The impact was stunning.

Today, many months later, I am still haunted by the aura of these places, and by questions unanswered. Something is missing. With all that grandiose space-age technology, there exists an inexplicable hollowness. Something intangible. What *is* this factor? I wonder, could "what-ever-it-is" be faulted for offsetting some of the benefits of emergency care? I will examine this but must first describe my impressions of an ICU as slowly they came into focus.

Upon entering the unit one senses a whirl of activity. At intervals I was permitted to watch as staff "worked" my spouse. He was suctioned, swabbed, scanned, manacled, monitored, radiated, respirated, hydrated, x-rayed, "electroded" and oxygenated. No stone, nor my spouse, was left unturned.

The *smells* of an ICU? Alcohol, antiseptics, blood, urine, disinfectants, sprays, deodorizers. The *sounds*? The beep-beep of monitors, pfft-pfft of respirators, clicks of x-rays, swoosh of cleaning pans, the drips, buzzes, clinks, clanks of instruments, the whht-whhts of sphygmomanometers. And the *human sounds*? Sighs, groans, yells, cries, calls, whispers of bedfast bodies.

Observing my husband I wonder how any three-fold (mind-body-spirit) creature can assimilate such a scene. Is he conscious? Can he sense the surroundings? Is he aware of his body, wired like a switchboard, fettered like a felon, punctured with plastic tubes which, like tentacles of an octopus, protrude from every orifice? Is he still a human being or a robot — an extra-terrestrial whose feelings are irrelevant to those who minister to him?

Throughout his ordeal I expect to stay by his side to comfort, encourage, smooth his forehead, hold his hand. But no. I am expendable. Soon after entering I am hustled out of his cubicle.

"But I am his wife," I protest. "He needs me."

"Sorry, Mrs. Fox. If there is any change, we'll call you."

My visits were limited to the first five minutes of each hour. For seventeen hours in the lounge I sweated, agonized, not knowing what was happening. Too tired, too numb to protest further. My own husband — how *could* they?

Preoccupied with technical details, staff is trained to consider superfluous any benefits a spouse may provide for the patient's morale. Throughout the night my family and I keep our vigil, mostly apart from my beloved. Each time I re-enter the unit, a new shock tears at my sensibilities.

In an adjoining cubicle I hear shufflings. A safari of interns gathers for daily rounds, all gung-ho, it seems, for capturing an "exciting" disgnosis. (Will they concede it's a *person* on that bed?) Sounds like they're deploying his body as a punching bag to prod, palpate, peek at, poke at his collections of "fascinating" symptoms. Picture the expressions on the students' faces as finally a suspected malfunction is identified for, as with hyenas capturing a cadaver, the catterwauling commences. Now the drape is pulled aside. I steal a peek. Delightedly flapping their wings, like crows they caw-caw. Eureka! A major medical breakthrough?

I keep wondering. What is that patient thinking, if he *can* think? Something like this? "Yea, team! I've always dreamed of owning the lucky body blessed with "Thoracic Outlet Compression Syndrome" or "Ventricular Fibrillation" or whatever, just so I could enchant and enthrall the medics! Who knows. If my luck holds out I may get to go to surgery for a spectacular choperation!"

Suddenly in that cubicle it's quiet. With a jab of another needle, the torso transcends to Tranquilsville. The medics move on.

Now I peek into another cubicle where another patient is being exposed to the conditioned reflexes of scientific teamwork. Well, I'm no doctor. But I wonder. Will she become yet another victim to exist solely on a biological level — her brain so blah, her physical function so stunted that, "thanks" to modern technology she'll be doomed to life as a vegetable? But the larger question: "Why, in our society (with the exception of those who plead for the holistic or mind-body-spirit approach to health care) is biological existence, per se, of supreme value? *Is not the physical body, unless sanctified by the indwelling mind and spirit, but a bag of bones?*.

That respirator, that intravenous tube — standard equipment, yes, but *must* they be used routinely even when life-saving becomes no more than delaying action to drag out the process of dying? Of prolonging agony?

And oh, the fiendish cost of it all! See that other patient over there, soon to take his final breath? (One hour later he expires.) But, at the eleventh hour, into his cubicle rolls the gigantic X-ray machine. "Gang-way everybody," calls the technician. I hop

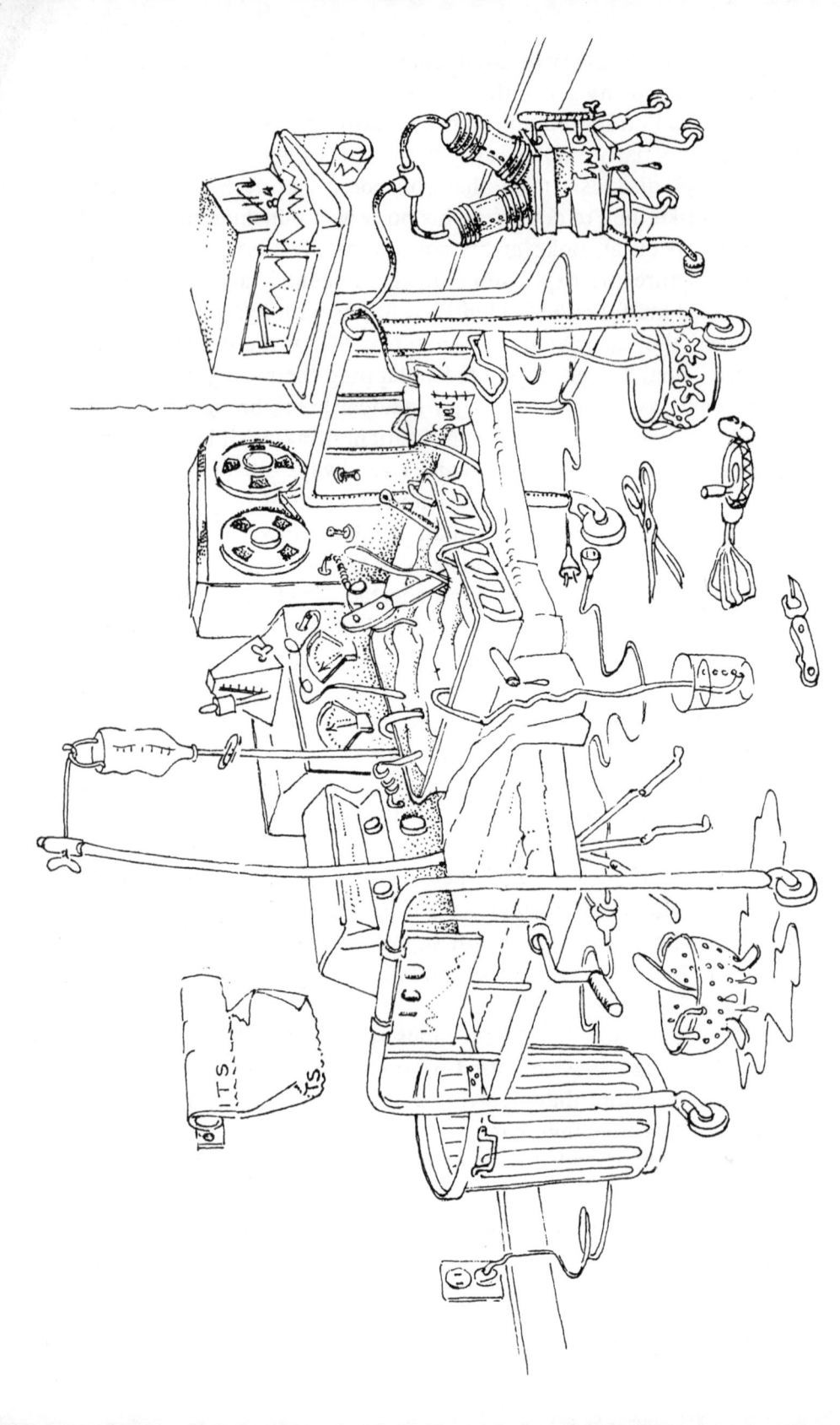

aside. "We need a picture of his lungs."

"*WE*" need it?" And who, may I ask, is "we?" For God's sake, this man is dying. He's practially dead. (How much did that X-ray job add to the final cost of his care? And if this photo of that lung is to be hung for research purposes on the laboratory wall-of-fame, then shouldn't the hospital pay the family of the deceased — pay them handsomely for the privilege?)

Yes, the American ICU leads the world, so we're told, in elaborate, costly technology. And yes, in many of these places one can find expert body care coupled with compassion and the caring touch. My spouse certainly got some of that. But the way ICU's are set up it is difficult if not impossible to stress the human side of emergency care. We've all seen how health care can be turned into assembly-line business; how bodies are rolled down the conveyor-belt of conformity.

No question. Today's ICU is a miracle. Lose a few, save a few lives. Loving, caring, dedicated, loyal professionals and paraprofessionals perform sensational feats of skill. Still, ethical questions persist, questions which must be confronted because I believe that today, the American public is disenchanted with medicine as practiced in the ICU. Laypersons find it topheavy, so science-oriented that it loses sight of the patient as an entity. We must therefore ask some hard questions of the medical profession as a whole, the individual doctor and nurse as well. Tell me:

Since it is known that even the comotose patient can be spiritually aware; can even discern the whisperings of staff, could you place more emphasis on safeguarding the sensibilities of your patients? Soften the surroundings? Could you at times minimize the sounds, the scurrying about? Further, to make these places more comforting, what about quiet background music, known to relieve tension? Why not reconsider that cold, unsightly — in fact monstrously scary equipment which envelops — rather, *devours* the patient? Terrifying! Surely through other dimensions of technology there must exist some creative ways to make the ICU more shock-proof. Through new design, perhaps, or disguise? (Kitchen appliances and car instruments are hidden or streamlined by recessing them into walls or dashboards.) Your expertise is there. Could you stand back and rethink the whole ICU concept *from the patient's point of view*?

And doctors, something else. Here I am really perplexed. As the cliche says, "Rules are rules," but when considering visitors, what about flexibility? For sure, the hysterical one has to go. But couldn't a designated staff person decide selectively who might remain at the bedside? (In your business you're pretty good judges of character.) You've seen the loving, controlled spouse — that dynamic force for healing and good morale who, with the loved one in crisis, establishes a spiritual bond surpassing what medicine can do? At a time when the victim walks a life-death tight-rope, must you cast his loved one aside? No, a thousand times no, if *you* were to be the victim and, in your crucial hour, *your* beloved was barred from your bedside!

Because I was sensitized by my husband's crisis, I now enter my plea to the medical and nursing staffs. If the time comes when the emergency is mine, do for me what you did for him. But only a part. Wheel me into the unit. Give me the same attention. I'll be grateful for your expertise and for the "fantastic" equipment at hand. But, as the hours pass and I linger on; if it is evident that I won't "make it," please *know when to stop*. Get me out of that madhouse of machines — that spiritually deadening horror-chamber. Get me home, even if this shortens my life a few hours or days. (My family knows what I want — they won't sue you!) Spare me further exposure to the tyranny of too much technology.

In familiar surroundings, put me in the haven of my own home. Let me die in the presence of those I love. Let my family ease me over the threshhold, not for just five minutes but, rotating their vigil, for all sixty minutes of each hour. At the end, let my loved ones see me, not as a mechanized mannequin; not as a zonked-out zombie, but as "good old Mah," wrapped in her sleazy bathrobe — the Mah they can touch and hug without a permit from the Board-of-Health. Let my grandkids climb on the bed, stroke my hair as firsthand they learn important lessons of life — *lessons that all ICU's deny to all children.* Allow my little Colby and Jenny to learn that dying is the natural culmination of living; that a leaf falls to make room for another leaf; that "Mima" has had her turn, and now is making way for a new baby being born somewhere out there in the world.

As I lie there, scrap the laws of sanitation. Bring in "China

Girl," my Siberian Husky. Let her put her white paw on my bed, let her lick my hand. Tell her I'll be waiting "up there" with her special ground-liver treat! And let my silky tabby cat, "Tabbyoca" and my Persian "Fuzzball" cuddle my neck, their soft inner motors emitting such comforting sounds.

Give me my inherent right to part from my loved ones, not as a stranger, not as a motorized inmate of a modern ICU, but as myself, "Mah," who wants (sans benefit of suction tubes) to tell my family: "God it was good to have you dear ones for so long!" And if I can't say it they will read in my eyes the gratitude I feel, the joys we have shared. And they will learn that life goes on; that "they are not dead who live in hearts they leave behind."

Dr. Paul Tournier, the Swiss physician, asks: "What kind of eyes does a patient see upon awakening? Are they eyes of love and concern or are they cold and impersonal? What kinds of arms and hands care for and lift the patient? Is the atmosphere that surrounds him one of warmth and serenity?" May our ICUs reflect this ideal.

Finally, to pose the ultimate question. "How can we, as a civilized, progressive nation, pay honor to each patient as a human being of dignity and worth?" With every ounce of your expertise, you good men and women of Medicine, can you not — or rather, *will you* find some way to *humanize* the American Intensive Care Unit?

*Just what does the U.S. want for her mentally impaired?*

## CHAPTER TWO

## CALL TO ARMS

## A Call to Arms

Sprawled on the floor, the near-naked old man is really no bother. "We just walk around him," murmurs the nursing aide as she shuffles her pack of cards. "That's Gus. He's lived here for years."

I walk past Gus, glance back, try to hide my dismay. "Same with Arthur, we hardly notice him anymore — we're used to him," continues the aide, noting my concern for a teenager who is circling the table. Increasing his pace, running ever more furiously, Arthur clutches his head as if to contain, within his brain, an unbearable buildup of pressure.

Hardly notice him? With those bulging eyes, that vacant stare? Wait a minute. You, the reader and the sensitive care-giver would notice him — you'd seek immediate help. The public would notice him if, outside of visiting hours, they could see what else is taking place within these walls.

I'm told there are nurses here, but none is in sight. Just the aide, "a high school dropout," she tells me. Bored, she plays solitaire, hardened to the suffering around her — the loneliness, the despair — she's neither motivated nor properly trained to deal with heavy challenge.

Now a shrill shriek. Then a crash. Abruptly the absent staff awakes from apathy. They come running from out of the woodwork. Now, oh yes, *now* they notice young Arthur.

Arthur has dropped dead.

### Where Are You, Staff?

These are some of the sights I saw — not in Outer Mongolia jails, not in a sixteenth century snake pit, but here, in progressive America. In numerous psychiatric hospitals.

Hoping to disprove popular rumors about these places, I began investigating. I had to convince myself that in today's institutions, with research and stress on human rights, psychiatric patients receive respect, holistic care as human beings of dignity and worth. However, with exceptions, this was not the case. I saw patients in physical and emotional despair. I saw too many apathetic, robot-like nurses. I saw top-sergeant tactics employed to "deal with" these unfortunates.

Because we can do better, I share my concern with you, the public, and with you in the health care field. Nurses, therapists, doctors, psychiatrists, administrators, social workers and volunteers in every department have much to offer these people. This is your challenge — to bring about change, to contribute to a mission possible.

### Despair and Degradation

Come with me into a large, barracks-like room, crowded with dejected men. In a corner two patients wallow in their own filth. The heat is stifling. Here, the patient comes last, for air conditioning is reserved for offices of doctors and administration. Perched overhead in this "gang-room" is a TV set, the picture doing a perpetual flip-flop. The sole "decor" is a hard bench which encircles the four walls. High up near the ceiling one small window lets in what light there is. No view to the outside. No curtains, pictures, flowers or plants. No proper lighting, no comfortable chairs. And, as in a heavy fog, the density of cigarette smoke reduces visibility to near zero, causing incessant coughing and hacking.

In a far corner a man slugs another. They lock in a stranglehold. Hearing the commotion, the "guard" pokes his head in the door. Amused, he withdraws.

My heart pounds. Angry tears block my vision. One of these inmates could be your uncle, brother, or my next-of-kin.

Hurriedly I exit to the quiet world of the outdoors — that world of beautifully manicured lawns which, apparently, is unknown to many patients.

In these places, is "holistic" (mind-body-spirit) care practiced with any degree of seriousness? Are not these persons worth our effort? Does not today's literature emphasize TLC, activities, therapy for the treatment of any illness, mental or physical? Why, then, do so few receive the advantages these measures can provide?

What about touch? The kind I saw was *rough* touch. Pushing, shoving — staff to inmate, inmate to inmate. And when it was inmate to staff, the "culprit" was marched off to "total security."

What about the "I care about you" approach? The daily backrub, the soft music to sooth the restless mind? And, to raise the rock-bottom self-esteem among patients, where is evidence of careful grooming? Look at that fellow in the torn jacket, run-down heels, stubbly facial growth. Why not more of a semblance of "gracious" dining rather than those ear-splitting sounds from the kitchen — the dish-clattering — enough to stretch already taut nerves to the limit. And what is the therapeutic benefit of long, cafeteria-style lines where hungry patients wait to be served by those who simply *slop* the food on their plates?

A dining room can be pleasing, with soothing decor in colors that invite congeniality. And here, especially, soft background music could make a difference in moods. Perhaps one could say that *without* these kinds of innovative approaches to mental health care, our system actually encourages mental and physical ill-health, magnifying the problems, driving away would-be new employees, contributing to that everlasting hiring-firing-quitting marathon which has come to be an accepted fact of life in many institutions.

Researchers tell us that our mental hospitals are filled with patients who do not now have, or never did have a meaningful one-to-one relationship with anyone. And so, another question: How much care is taken to orient volunteers and families to fill this void? How much time is provided for reality orientation, time for stretching horizons with pets to love, young people to visit and play games? What percentage of patients gets the chance to absorb

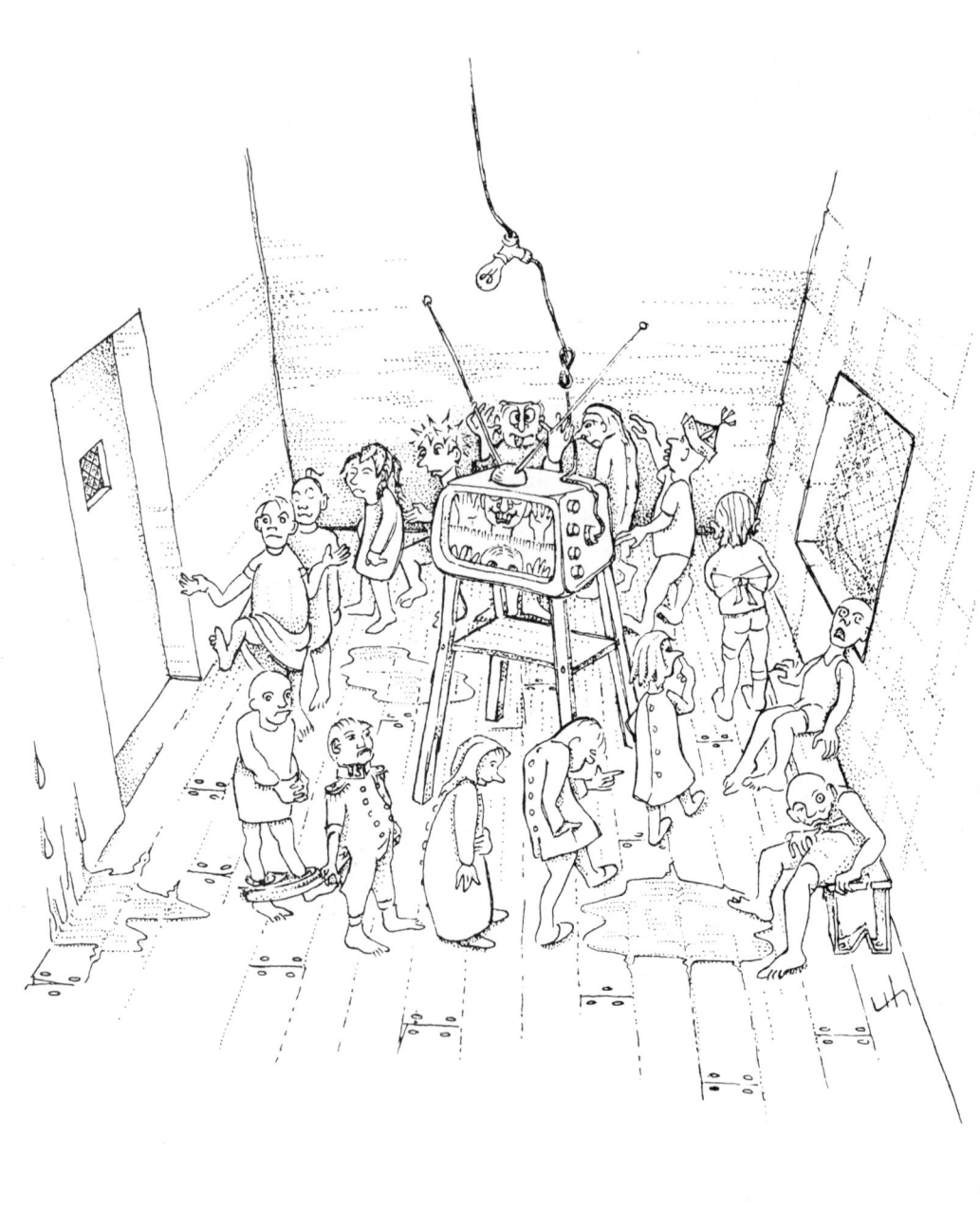

the beauties of nature, or to enjoy horticultural therapy? *Too much time within four walls deadens the spirit.*

I see a group of patients making leather belts. But why so few — just a handful amoung hundreds of residents. Couldn't occupational therapy, with its manual labor, its creative outlets displace, to a large degree, the obsession with cigarettes? "All the conversation I get around here," said one man lolling on a bench, is: "Got a weed, Bud?"

### Short of Time, Short of Staff?

Who, may I ask, inspects these institutions? Show me their qualifications. What are their standards, their attitudes towards human beings in general, the mentally ill in particular?

No, I'm not suggesting luxury or pampering. I'm talking about essentials for the human spirit — those essentials that embrace warmth and trust, the reaching towards the highest potential of mind, body and soul for each person here in residence. What one sees permeating the place, however, is an attitude of hopelessness.

"All that you suggest," said a staff member to me, "is fine and dandy. Sure, but no time." To that, an administrator adds: "And besides, we're always short of help."

To which I reply: "No time? Horsefeathers! Look around. Staff stands around in clusters, talking endlessly among themselves. Staff loiters in nursing stations not doing business-related work. Staff finds adequate time, however, to scold, play cards, avoid patients, watch the clock for check-out time."

But not *all* staff. I did see some who do well despite horrendous lack of cooperation by other staff; despite negative attitudes all around. When their task is difficult, back-breaking, heart-breaking, all power to them. They retain their sense of mission. But we question the qualification of bored aides and orderlies, depressed nurses, invisible doctors, administrators who are wedded to their computers and calculators — worlds away from wards and the everyday woes.

Can a patient improve with none, or at very least a minimum of therapy and counseling? We do know this. That they haven't a prayer if no attempt is made to give an individual meaningful attention of some kind or another on a daily basis. Is custodial care the best they can expect? Where is the linkup of holistic theory and practice in the care of our mentally ill?

### Enter the Supernurse, the Trained Volunteer

Good people, you are needed — you with your courage to protest, your initiative to revive morale, your belief in TLC. If challenge is your bag, apply for work in a psychiatric hospital. You can make a difference as your attitude influences staff, right up the hierarchial ladder.

Lonely, fearful and inwardly tearful, the psychiatric patient is trapped in the morasses of his own mind. Touch, love, a listening ear — these are the drugs he most needs, yet rarely receives. Take Saul, for example.

Like most persons, Saul responds to a loving approach, retarded though he may be. We saw clear evidence, during the following episode of how TLC and how respect for him as a person made a difference. "Big Saul" was six foot three, a veritable King Kong of a man. Barging out of his room, he rushed towards the head nurse. Frantic, she bolted down the corridor, grabbed on to my waist, crouched behind me.

You couldn't blame her. Big Saul was bad news. And now, tearing after her, he was blocked. In that split second I thought: "What's my most powerful weapon? Fear? No." Though scared silly, I made eye contact with him. "Saul," I cried, "we love you. You wouldn't hurt us. Here, take my hand. We're friends!"

Screeching to a stop, Saul stepped backwards, relaxed his clenched fists, dropped his arms. Gently we led him back to his room. Relieved, he blurted: "I didn't mean it — I really didn't." We gave him his medication. Not the usual kind, but an even more effective tranquilizer, the infallible "Hug-drug!" Saul grinned.

### A National Dilemma

Remember the song: "What Lola Wants, Lola Gets?" Whatever America wants, too, America gets. Just what does the U.S. want for her mentally ill? Mere existence or a better life? Are we satisfied to herd them into stockyards where dependency, conformity and apathy are the rule? Content to ignore human deterioration where, in most cases, it can be salvaged? If this is what America wants *she's getting what she wants.* And at enormous cost in anguish to patients and their families; in wasted lives; in disgrace upon our society and in mind-boggling cost to taxpayers.

Step forward, caregivers and volunteers. Heed the call. Seek work in your local, state or other psychiatric hospitals. Be a missionary to the mentally ill. Match theory with practice. Keep aflame your social conscience. The plight of one American is the plight of us all.

You are a powerful channel through whom change can be initiated.

"But," you say, "I am only one."

Yes, but you *are* one! Stand tall and be counted. Make that Pledge of Allegiance come to life. This is One Nation, indivisible, under God, with Liberty and Justice — not just for some — not just for the mentally well — but for *all.*

*"Without care of the emotions, there is no cure for the body."*
*Socrates*

## CHAPTER THREE

## VISIBLE VS. INVISIBLE NURSING

## Visible vs. Invisible Nursing

"Students, don't judge yourselves by what the patient thinks!"

So we were taught by a nursing instructor who added: "If Mr. Jones in Room 68 says: 'You're the greatest!' or, if Mrs. Smith rejects you, ignore them both. After all, a patient cannot tell a good nurse from a poor one. Let staff do the judging."

I remembered that warning years later when two nurses locked horns in a geriatric ward. The first, Jean, agreed with the philosophy. On the job she was highly visible, hustling and bustling. A "hard worker," she was slated for promotion. Her patients, however, disliked her aloof manner. The second nurse, Norma, although she completed her assignments, never seemed to be "working her head off." Often she would vanish behind closed doors, becoming invisible as she heard out an anguished patient. Her patients adored her for the emotional support she provided. Whenever she did this, "Aha," complained her colleagues, "Norma's goofing off again!"

Never mind what the patient thinks? Surely this notion is due for an overhaul. If the patient is the primary concern of the staff, then his feelings *do* matter.

Still another wall separated Jean from Norma. Taking literally that "don't get involved" dictum," Jean maintains a rigid professional stance; doesn't care what patients think or feel. But Norma, upon observing the loneliness, the losses, the depression many patients experience, rebutts this theory of non-involvement. "Mush," she says. "Do get involved. To the extent that you are able; to the extent that you maintain you own equilibrium; to the extent that you do not encourage dependency, *get involved*. Or be a robot."

How did these two nurses fare professionally? Fascinated, I stood by and watched. Jean hit the heights, became charge-nurse and then, Director of Nursing Services. Norma remained in the ranks. Inevitably, retaining their differing views, the two women collided. Norma tells how it happened:

"Jean caught me redhanded — discovered my arms around Mrs. Watson who, despondent, was mourning a loss. For me it was too much. My own eyes filled with tears. Just as the patient was calming down, like a crack of lightning came Jean's curt command. 'Norma, come at once to my office.'

"As I stood before the 'Judge,' Jean errupted full blast. 'Never — do you hear, Norma, don't you ever again shed a tear or show emotion on the job or, I warn you, *you'll never make it as a nurse!*' "

Norma recalls another time when she "failed" her boss. A patient had just died. Staff scurried back to assigned duties. Norma, however, remained in the room to comfort the weeping relatives. Escorting them out to their car, she kept her arms around the distraught daughter of the deceased woman. Helping her into the car, Norma said: "We loved your mother. We'll miss her. Do think of us as your friends, and visit us sometime, won't you? In your great sorrow we will remember you."

As Norma walked back towards the front portal, there, adamant, with hands on hips, stood the Director of Nursing. "Norma," she fired, "goofing off again?"

Norma was becoming discouraged. "Not too many days would pass," she told me, "that I was not reprimanded for my actions in caring for patients." And I ached for her as she related another episode.

"I'll never forget," she said. "It was Christmas Eve. I was helping Mrs. Barnes to bed. Together we were humming carols. She

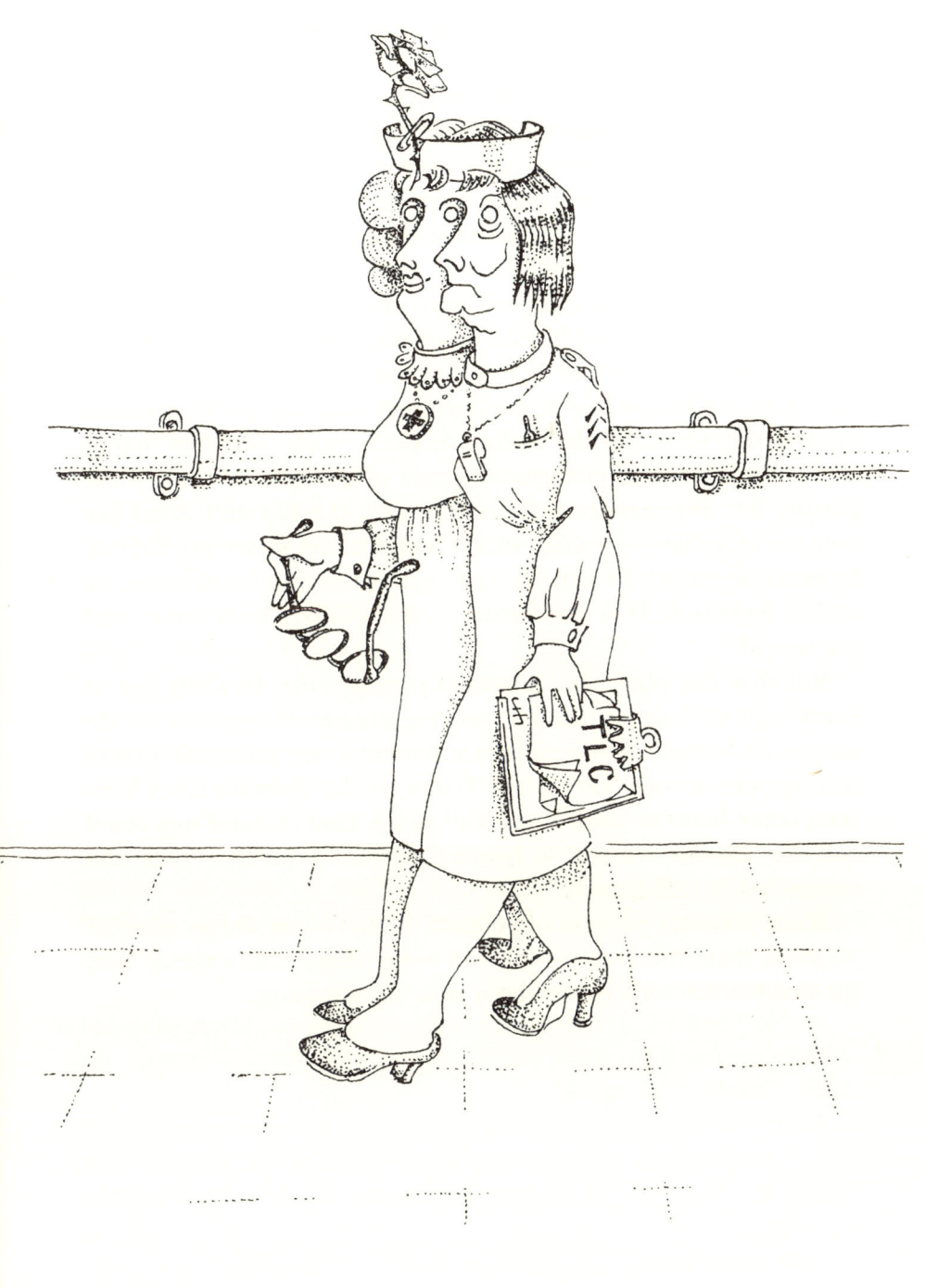

asked me if it were snowing and I told her it was coming down gently. 'Norma,' she said, 'just once again I would so love to feel the snow in my hands.'

"Helping her into the wheelchair, I took her to the lobby where she waited as I ran outside, scooped up a handful of snow and brought it to her. She was so happy and went back to bed, relishing memories of other Christmases with her family. That night she died in her sleep. I was reprimanded because 'we don't have extra time like that for patients.' "

As time passed, Norma pondered these encounters with her "boss." The more she did, the more her own feelings solidified. And today, secure in her belief that the holistic approach is the *only* way, she knows that in nursing, high visibility (or the medical model) only scratches the surface of client needs. She sees that to live is to experience continuous stages of growth and that, while putting her experiences into perspective, she has cultivated her own set of values — values which now she can staunchly defend. Norma's approach to patient care rejects the non-involvment, or visible approach. It is ineffectual. It demoralizes both server and the served.

Not that she plays the "angel-of-mercy" role, freaking out at every sign of distress. Rather, seeking greater recognition of the danger of bottled emotions in her patients, she promotes shared feelings, one-to-one encounters. Today, as she observes other Normas, other Jeans at work — as well as the kind of nurse one could call the "Double Nurse," (a healthy merger of the two types) she comes to this conclusion:

When you dare not give of yourself — that is, the deeper parts of yourself, then, it is true — you will never make it as a nurse. Nor, for that matter, will you make it as a human being.

**PART TWO:** *NURSING HOMES*
A Generation in Jeopardy?

**CHAPTER 4**

**IS THIS "SENILITY" NECESSARY?**

# Is This "Senility" Necessary?*

### A. "INFANTIZING"

"Cutie, it's time to go potty-chair!"
"Are we ready for our little pill, Ducky?"
"Here, let's put on our bib, shall we?"

These comments are samples of "infantizing," that is, the pressuring of an institutionalized adult into a state of infancy. This is the first of three practices that robs him of identity, of self-esteem and contributes to mental decline. It induces what I call "man-made senility."

While only a small percentage of the elderly suffer incurable, irreversible brain damage, (including those nearly two million diagnosed with Alzheimer's disease) countless others fall prey to preventable, reversible confusion of mind. Torsos tilting sideways, eyes glassy, mouths drooling — do you think that in old age these symptoms are inevitable?

In a federal study on long term care, surveyors noted that in many facilities, patients' dependency attitudes were constantly reinforced by the manner in which staff addressed them, often as

---

*Originally published by "The Oregonian," Jan. 1980. To this day the conditions described remain the rule, rather than the exception in U.S. nursing homes.

though speaking to a child. Mrs. Amy Park, whose tragic story is told in chapter eight, can tell you about "infantizing."

A dress protector is tied around her neck, only they call it a "bib." She keeps hearing words like "diapers," "honey-child," and wonders when they will hand her a rattle or chuck her under the chin with a giggly "goo-goo-ga-ga!" Simply because of diminished sight and poor health, she has been stripped of her adult status, molded into a miniature of her former self.

"Treat me like a child, call me 'Cutie,' " exclaims her roommate, "and I will stamp my feet and throw my food on the floor. But then, you can't win. People will call me 'senile.' "

Across the hall Mr. Pruitt tosses in the night. He longs for a glass of warm milk but this time he won't ring his call bell. He can't forget the response he got the last time. Said the nursing assistant: "If we'd eaten our din-din last night we wouldn't be so hungry now, would we?"

But Mr. McGuire tackles the "opposition" headon. Into his room trips the new little aide. "Are we ready for our bath?" she squeals. "YES," bellows the disgusted old gentleman, "*WE* are ready. *Let's* jump in!"

Sick of being babied, Mr. Hardy's tactics for resistance are slightly irregular. On his bed he lies stark naked. Every morning you can count on it — covers, pajamas piled on the floor. Staff walks in, scowls, walks out. Mr. Hardy smirks. "That'll fix 'em!" Considering themselves experts at instant diagnosis, employees label him "senile, childish, dirty-old man." For our strip-teaser it's the old "shame-on-you, you-naughty-naughty-boy" approach. Staff is told: "Other than provide food and medications, just ignore him."

Granted this man's behavior is difficult. But to one nurse he seems alert, reasonably intelligent, certainly not "senile." Is he lonely, she wonders? Is he protesting our condescending approach? Then perhaps he needs more, rather than less attention. Proceeding on this premise, she enters his room, pulls up the covers and says: "Mr. Hardy, I see by your chart that you hail from the great state of Texas?"

No response. Mr. Hardy turns to the wall. "And that before retirement you taught biology?"

"Big deal. What do you care? Drop dead!"

Each day this nurse repeats the procedure, varying her questions and conversation. Finally, though suspicious of her sincerity, Mr. Hardy reacts. He begins to talk. He moans of his past failures, of his children who never visit, of his divorce. Here, masked by melodramatics, is a thinking feeling human being, starved for meaningful relationships.

In time, aides enter his room to find him fully dressed, talking with his roommate. Staff learns to accept and appreciate him. They bring him science books from the library and track down a fellow biologist from the local high school who becomes a regular visitor. In return, Mr. Hardy reads to bedfast patients, waters plants, pushes wheelchairs. Formerly afraid of him, staff now may be seen, their arms around him, walking together down the hall.

In despair, Mr. Hardy had uncovered his body. But when the staff uncovered his heart and mind; when they conversed with him adult-to-adult, they discovered the real Mr. Hardy, the man he had always been, a human being of dignity and worth.

### B. Too Much Rest

The second contributor to "man-made senility" is called, quite simply, "rest."

"Rest?" you exclaim. "Come now. What's wrong with rest? We all need it."

Would you believe that rest, this seemingly harmless pastime, can demoralize a person if taken in too large doses? It's that "you-need-your-rest" syndrome, sanctioned by too many "rest" homes. Too much — no end of rest.

Gerontologists generally agree that one of the most dangerous treatments for the elderly is enforced inactivity. (This applies, in fact, to persons of any age.) Yet the average nursing home promotes passivity and immobility which can and do lead to total disability.

"Nonsense," you protest, "they have activity programs galore — the law requires it."

Yes, but take a count. What percentage of clients actually participate in activities at all? And how many do this on a daily basis? How many residents sit in the halls for hours on end, staring at walls?

"Nonsense again," you insist. "Nobody ever died of rest."

Oh no? If he could, the late Mr. Carr would disagree with you. What happened to him happens to far too many shut-ins. Arriving at the home, he is introduced to his roommate and to the staff. After that, not much communication, for repeatedly he is told: "Time to rest. Doctor's orders." And so he gets it. Plenty of rest. Mornings he lolls on his bed. Afternoons he dozes in his chair. Evenings, he's put to bed at a child's early hour. After only one week, Mr. Carr begins to see for himself a bleak future.

Months pass. Lack of physical and mental stimulation take their toll. His interest in life drained, Mr. Carr now qualifies for the "Seniles Club." He forgets easily. Mumbles to himself. Bladder and sphincter control gone, he soils himself, gets frequently scolded. Time now to join that catheterized, bed-ridden, faceless throng, victims of the "plenty-of-rest" school of thought. Soon he develops a bladder infection, then bedsores. Not surprisingly, he is hospitalized for pneumonia, suffers transplantation shock. Totally confused. His latest medical orders? You guessed it. "Plenty of rest!"

"Yes," agrees the staff, "he needs his rest."

Three days later he gets the best rest there is, the most perfect rest known to "man." He's resting in peace. A sheet is pulled over his head.

Positive that they have provided tender loving care, unaware of mismanagement, the medical and nursing staffs make the standard comment: "Oh, well, Harry's better off now. Nothing to live for!"

Perhaps you, the reader, have an inkling what happens to minds and bodies when all this resting goes on, even though health professionals often forget that this can trigger:

> Dulling of the intellect
> Metabolic imbalances
> Increased dependency
> Circulatory deterioration
> Mental confusion
> Lack of sensory stimulation
> Loss of muscular strength
> Loss of bone calcium
> Deterioration of the cerebro-vascular system
> and finally,
> Loss of self-esteem and will to live.

Although today many physicians and nurses are cutting down on those interminable rest periods, they are often opposed by other staff members or relatives of the patient who complain: "Why change his routine? Old people have worked hard all their lives — they deserve their rest!"

### C. Dangerous Tranquility

The third contributor to "man-made senility" is a drug — that medically prescribed tranquilizer.

The next time you visit a nursing home, extend your antennae. With eyes, ears, and nose, tune in — don't just observe, *scrutinize* the place. Peek into remote corners. Take the elevator to the top floors where certain "hopeless" patients may be stashed away, out of sight, out of the public mind. In some homes, especially in large cities, what do you find? Patients not recognizing their families. Heads flopping into supper trays. Bodies tied to chairs. Voices mumbling, cackling, wailing, screaming. Of course, ravaging diseases such as advanced Alzheimer's can cause these conditions. But, barring those, our immediate concern is: How many of these unfortunates are paying the penalty of months, even years of mismanagement? How many were "infantized," over-rested, over-sedated? We ask the burning question: *"Is this senility necessary?"*

According to one estimate, over one hundred million dollars worth of tranquilizers are used yearly in U.S. nursing homes. They put people in a position where they won't complain or expect service. And it's a fine way to hasten "senility."

Jails are filled with political prisoners. Many of our elders, too, living in jails of their own, are prisoners of altered states of consciousness. Says Dr. Alexander Simon, (for years the medical director of Langley-Porter Neuro-Psychiatric Institute in San Francisco): "Once you start giving any kind of sedative medication that has an effect on the metabolism of the brain, you may precipitate an acute confusional state, especially likely in aged patients. This can easily be mistaken for senility."

For every drug consumed, there are side effects. Each new one added increases the potential for reaction. And so, what about *reactions* which are treated by adding *more* drugs? Consider this ad, placed in professional journals: "If drug-induced Parkinsonism threatens to interrupt tranquilizer therapy, just add — (drug name withheld). A pyramid. One drug atop another ad infinitum.

Now you and I are not doctors or pharmacologists, but neither are we dummies. Sometimes even the patient is aware of the lunacy of this sort of thing. He spits the stuff out!

This is not to deny the need and value of drugs for the elderly. Pharmacologist Edward Brady, M.S. describes his concern: "Drugs can stupify, injure, cause waste and harmful problems that could be prevented." Patients who take tranquilizers often suffer reactions which require hospitalization. As if that were not anguish enough, they experience additional drug reactions while in the hospital, often doubling their length of stay. For the elderly, hospitals can be dangerous places.

What part do drug companies play in the overall picture? A downright powerful part. They spend 630 million dollars a year on salesmen who peddle pills to physicians. That's twice the size of the FDA (Food and Drug Administration budget). The FDA is outspent, outnumbered, outmaneuvered by the industry it is supposed to control. Drug companies spend over two billion dollars a year to advertise* — a sum far greater than their expenditures for research and development.

Clever ads blur the judgment of many a physician, which appeal to "ease of management" or "social control," rather than to the therapeutic needs of patients. In bold red letters, a certain ad dramatizes the "tantrums" of a patient while, in 140 lines of tiny print, it mentions, as required by law, the possible adverse effects of this drug, ranging anywhere from jaw twitchings to toxic confusional states to sudden death. Other ads stress "reduction of work load" for the caregiver. And then, there's the one which accentuates the positive by depicting a winsome, brightly attired grandmother — oh so joyous, oh so relaxed, oh so sedated!

Because of physiological changes, the elderly cannot absorb drugs nearly as rapidly as younger persons. Side effects are more severe. Said Dr. Eric Pfeiffer of Duke University Medical Center: "We must be extraordinarily cautious in the use of drugs in the elderly who have delicately balanced systems which can easily be derailed by a number of drugs which have proved beneficial in younger persons."

*Report of House Select Committee on Aging, July, 1983. Publication #98-409

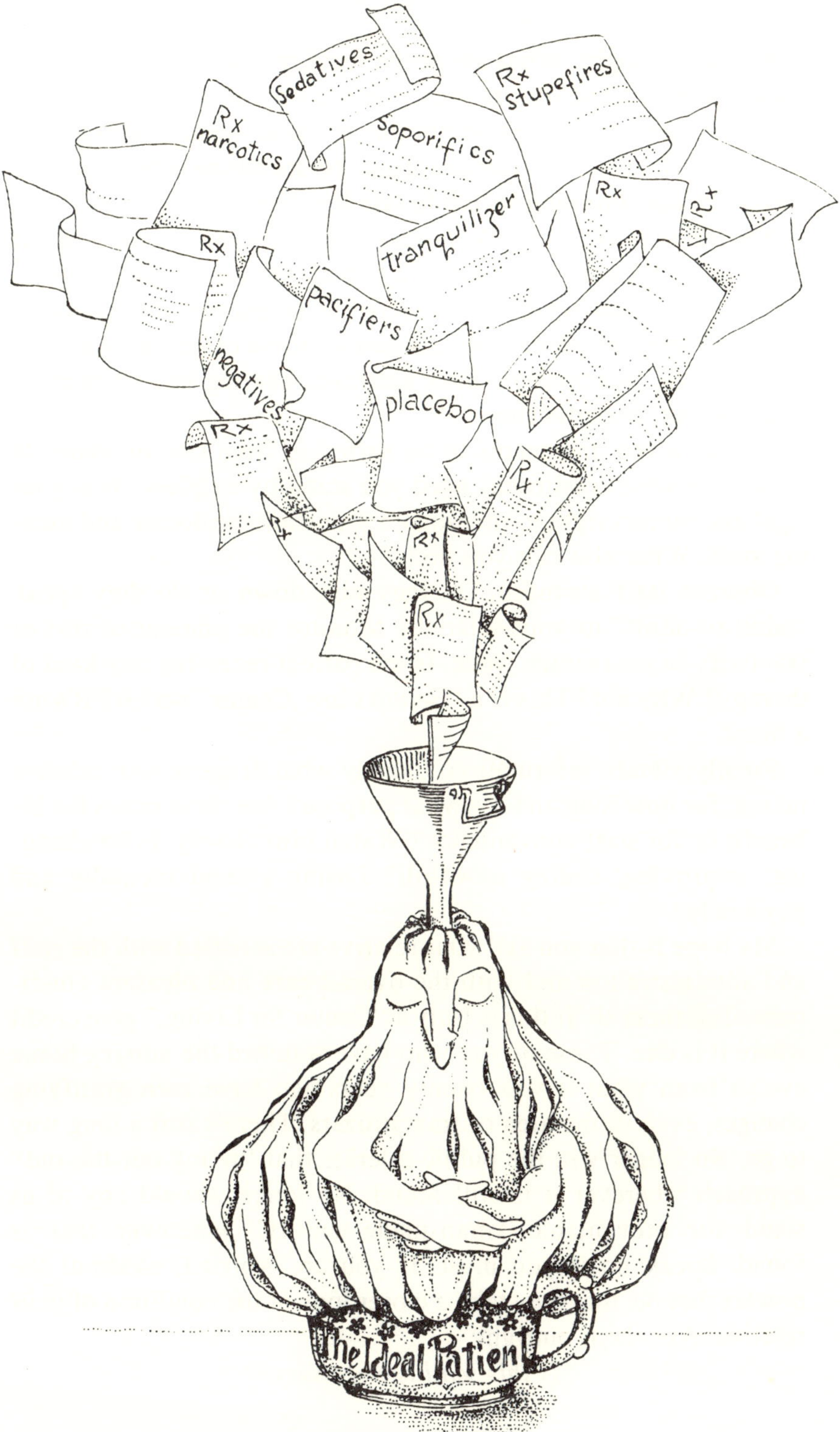
Sedatives
Rx
Stupefires
Rx
narcotics
Soporifics
tranquilizer
Rx
pacifiers
negatives
placebo
The Ideal Patien

Another thought. What about the legality of overdrugging? Excessive use of tranquilizers may infringe on patients' rights.

These, then, are three contributors to "man-made senility." Infantizing, over rest and over drugging. Torsos tilting sideways, eyes glassy, mouths drooling — *no*! In late life, these are not inevitable.

According to Dr. Mary Wolanin (voted the 1982 Gerontological Nurse of the Year) there are a hundred physiological causes of mental confusion which are reversible or preventable. (Not to mention the many psychological causes.) Some examples: Anemia, stress, drugs, constipation, poor nutrition, hearing loss, transplantation shock, hypertension.

If your loved one seems to be suffering from one or many of these reversible conditions, need you stand by helpless? It is your legal and human right to investigate. Question the doctor and nursing staff. What else can you do?

Observe staff attitudes. Do they talk down or do they speak "adult-to-adult" to your relative? Monitor the amount of rest or inactivity in an average week. Is the patient receiving any kind of therapy? Why not? This is a *"Health Care* Center" isn't it? It's *not* a hotel!

Finally, obtain information. Exactly what drugs is your relative taking, for how long and for what purpose? Are these drugs for his benefit or for staff convenience? Watch him closely. Is he changing, improving, sliding downhill? Losing ground mentally and physically?

My hope is that you and your relative are satisfied with the staff and administration and with the overall care and pleasant conditions. Tell them so. If this is truly a "Center for Living," give credit where it is due. Those of you who have watched the nursing home evolve from what it was twenty years ago have seen gratifying changes, even in the area of tranquilizers. There's still a long way to go. No longer will the public tolerate that "wring-out-the-old" approach wherever it is still found. No longer should any of us stand for preventable "man-made-senility" wherever that is found. Speak up if you must. If you are worried, confront the powers that be, that they take a closer look at the condition of your relative. Ask them outright:

*"Is this senility necessary?"*

*A not-so-funny whodunnit
"mellerdrammer"*

## CHAPTER FIVE

## MURDER BY NUTRITION, or . . .
## IT TAKES A CAST-IRON STOMACH!

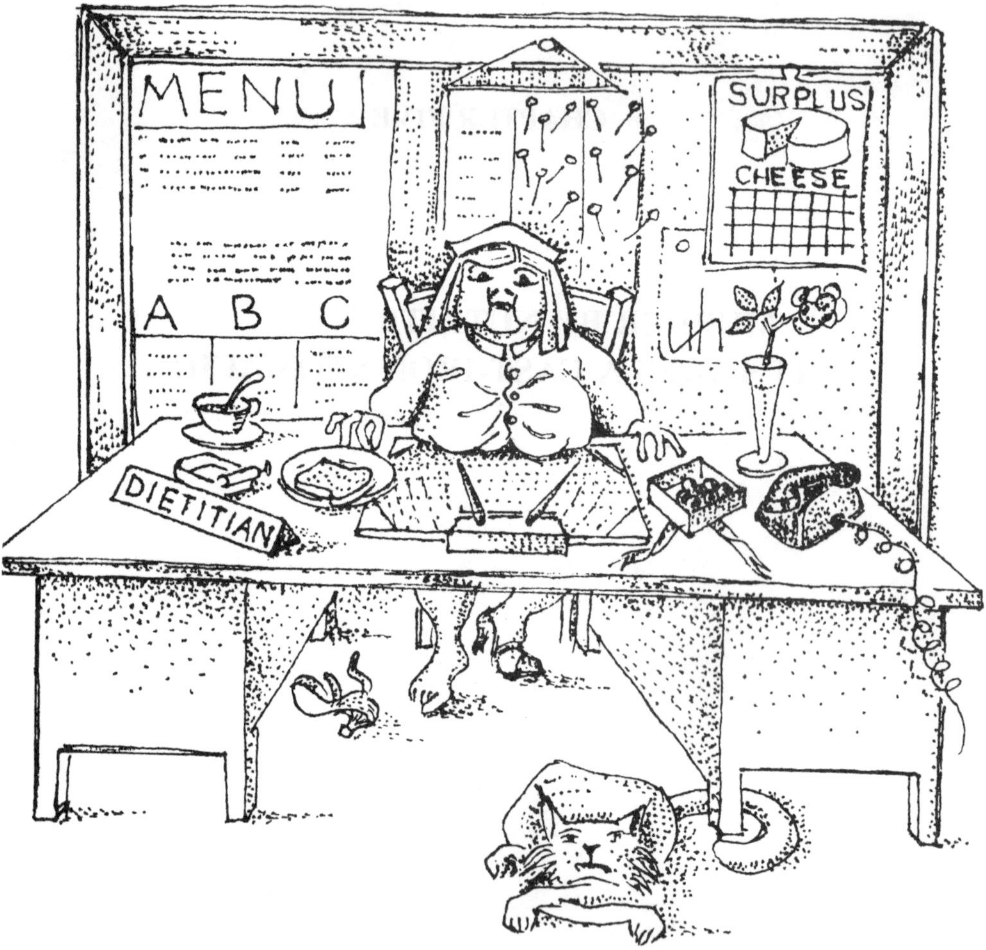
MENU
A B C
SURPLUS
CHEESE
DIETITIAN

*Minds, bodies, spirits are profoundly affected by the kind of food served in institutions. Too often it is the meal, rather than the patient's behavior, which should be analyzed!*

*Skip this chapter if the dietary department is adequately budgeted to provide wholesome, varied and eye-appealing meals.*

## *Murder by Nutrition*
### or,
## It Takes a Cast-Iron Stomach!

SETTING: "Sunhaven," a posh nursing home in Denver, or Anywhere.

CAST: Hilda, the Head Nurse
Mr. Dan, a sixty-year-old resident
The Kitchen Crew
O'Hara and Jones, Police Officers
Mr. Humboldt, Reporter from the *Denver Post*
Gabriel, the Guardian Angel

### Scene One
(Lunchtime)

**Nurse Hilda:** Now eat, Mr. Dan, it's good for you.
**Mr. Dan:** But Nurse, I'm not hungry. I feel punk.
**Nurse Hilda:** Come now, it's nutritious!
**Mr. Dan:** Who says so?
**Nurse Hilda:** (impatiently) Come on. Eat. EAT!
**Mr. Dan:** O.K. I'll eat. Even if it kills me!

**(IT KILLS HIM)**

## Scene Two
(Enter two police officers)

**O'Hara:** On with the investigation. Looks like murder. Strange, this Mr. Dan mystery! And of all places, too, this licensed, certifed, government-inspected facility, Colorado's poshest!

**Jones:** Oh, but a fancy facade can fool you. This could be one of those "fake-food facilities." Look here, O'Hara. (He pulls from his pocket a U.S. Senate report.) This says that institutional food ranks high in deficiencies.

**O'Hara:** Then quick! We'll comb the kitchen, the cook and all culinary department suspects.

(Frozen with fright, the kitchen crew cringes. Ransacking the place, the officers discover a top-secret document, posted on the wall. What could it be? Why, it's today's menu. (Perhaps a clue to Mr. Dan's demise?)

---
### MENU
### Sunhaven Care Center
#### BREAKFAST
Orange Juice, imitaion, yellow coloring
Milk, non-dairy
Toast, white (80% vitamins, minerals removed)
Eggs, artificial, chemically produced, yellow dye
Cereal, sugar-drenched, with BHA & Pyrodoxinehydrochloride
#### LUNCH
Wieners, sodium ascorbate, artificial flavor, red coloring
Potatoes, powdered, fake flavor
Green Beans, blanched, devitaminized, overcooked
Jello, offumaric acid, socium citrate, artificial color
Cake, acid phyrophosphate, Xanthan Gum, Polysorbste 80
#### DINNER
Beef Pie, monosodium glutamate, synthetic color, nitrites
Stove-top dressing, sulphur dioxide, tertiary butyhydroquinone, sodium nitrite
Cookies, sorbitan monostearate, synthetic sweeteners
Pudding, propoleneglycomonoesters, mono- and di-glycerides, fake flavor, brown dye

O'Hara: Great Scott! Mr. Dan was *polluted!* Another case of murder-by-nutrition. (With a menacing scowl he points an accusing finger at the scared-stiff staff and shouts:) YOU! WHEW! A demolition crew! Non-foods, fake-foods, junk-foods. Yikes! Why even . . .

Jones: . . . (rudely interrupting) . . . even a cast-iron stomach would corrode!
(THE CHEF SWOONS)

O'Hara: (ignoring the fallen chef) Looks like Mr. Dan is the latest victim of Nutrition, American Style.

Jones: Yeah. Something's rotten in Denver.

### Scene Three

(DASHING TO THE NURSES' STATION, THE TWO OFFICERS NAB NURSE HILDA AS SHE TRIES TO FLEE)

O'Hara: (Clicking on the handcuffs) Nurse, let's have it. Prior to your patient's collapse, any evidence of foul play?

Hilda: No, no, a thousand times no!

Jones: Methinks the lady protests too much!

O'Hara: (pounding his fist) Hilda, you're under oath.

Hilda: Well, uh . . . it's just that during Mr. Dan's ten weeks here, his skin had become scaley, bones soft, muscles flabby, mind muddled and plumbing clogged. No real evidence of foul play, except that his nine body systems (muscular, skeletal, excretionary, circulatory, sensory, endocrine, reproductive, digestive and respiratory) — they all just up-and-quit on him. What with his diet, drugs, laxatives unlimited, I *did* suspect foul play, actually, but Sirs, I *had to follow orders.* Doctor's orders.

Jones: What was Dr. Brown's diagnosis, upon Mr. Dan's admittance?

Hilda: Hangnail on left index finger. Otherwise, healthy as a horse.

**Jones:** What was the doctor's verdict as to cause of collapse?
**Hilda:** Died of natural causes. "What can you expect?" said the doctor, "It's his *age*."
**Jones and O'Hara:** (simultaneously) His AGE? HIS *AGE*? Why Mr. Dan was just a sixty-year-old kid.
(FLABBERGHASTED, THE OFFICERS EXIT SHOUTING)
*"The public must hear of this!"*

(MAKING A BEE-LINE FOR THE PHONE, THE COPS DIAL THE DENVER POST. REPORTER HUMBOLDT PICKS UP THE RECEIVER. THE WIRES CRACK, SIZZLE AND POP.)

### Scene Four
(In Sunhaven's Lounge)

(ENTER REPORTER HUMBOLDT. NOSTRILS TWITCHING LIKE A BLOODHOUND, HE CORNERS THE NORMALLY CALM BUT NOW HYSTERICAL HILDA, GRABS HER TO TRACK DOWN THE TRUTH.)

**Humboldt:** Now, Hilda, give it to me straight.
**Hilda:** First let go of me, you beast!
**Humboldt:** (unruffled) Sure, why not? I'm a peace-loving man. Now, Doll, first shall we dance?
**Hilda:** Cut the corn. Wanna know exactly how it was? O.K. Before he entered Sunhaven to convalesce from his hangnail, Mr. Dan was blooming with health — a fresh fruit and vegetable fan. He told me how he'd smacked his lips just from reading the Sunhaven menu. Say, here's what it says in the PR brochure. I'll read it to you.

"SUNHAVEN'S RENOWN CUISINE OFFERS DELICIOUS, WHOLESOME MEALS, PREPARED BY CULINARY EXPERTS. WE STRESS GOOD NUTRITION, BALANCED TO PERFECTION TO MAINTAIN THE HIGHEST PHYSICAL AND MENTAL STATUS OF OUR SUNHAVEN RESIDENTS."

Hilda: (continuing) Here's evidence. On the very day he was admitted to Sunhaven, I took this picture of Mr. Dan smacking his lips. However, within one week, he became pale and pasty. His pipes got clogged. So I phoned Dr. Brown. "Hmmmm Hmmmm," yawned the doctor, "so Danny-boy's pipes are calling — ho! ho! — calling a halt, that is. Now take this prescription. Mix two ounces of each ingredient and administer it to him every hour on the hour."

**RX: X-LACKS, LAXIBLAST, SEROOTAN, EXPLOSITAN, DYNAMITOSE, VALLYUM, FENOBARBIT OIL AND METTYMOOSAL**

... and so, Mr. Humboldt, I followed orders. Dutifully Mr. Dan downed his first dose, then, like a breeze, wafted benignly into Blahsville. But suddenly, eyes rolling, he shot up straight, emitted a volcanic roar and pfft! Like a house of cards, he collapsed, a rubbled heap on the floor. Dead as a doornail.

Humboldt: (bolting out the door) Thanks, Hilda. You *are* a doll! Whatta story for the *Evening Gossiptimes!* Murder-by-nutrition! Thanks one helluva lot. Wahoo!!

### Scene Five

(IN THE NEWSROOM OF THE DENVER POST, OUR REPORTER, FEET ON TABLE, CIGAR IN HAND, IS CONCLUDING HIS REPORT TO THE U.P. WIRES.)

Humboldt: ... and now, while Sunhaven's fake-food-and-drug administration is under criminal investigation, let this case remind us "civilized" Americans to take another look at those "backward," nature food lovers who to this day remain blissfully uncontaminated by Nutrition-American-Style.

(SLOWLY THE CURTAIN STARTS TO DESCEND)

# Epilogue

(MEANWHILE, UP AT THE HEAVENLY RANCH, WE GLIMPSE MR. DAN, OUR HALOED HERO, VIGOROUSLY FLAPPING HIS WINGS — (HIS NINE BODY SYSTEMS NOW BACK TO NORMAL, HE QUERIES HIS GUARDIAN ANGEL:)

**Mr. Dan:** Say, Gabriel, quit that horn and hear me out. Ever since my fatal Murder-by-Nutrition I've been wondering. Tell me. Could it be, after all, that the U.S. down there is *still* a backward, disadvantaged nation?

**Gabriel:** Good question. Let's get a concensus. Toot toot. (He summons his angels.)

Instantly, from his Heavenly host, there burst forth the sound of trumpets — a mighty "YEA," a thunderous "AMEN."

*That catch-all phrase, "Quality Care."
More than simply adherence to "codes,"
more than fancy decor, here is this author's
definition.*


CHAPTER 6


# WHO, ME? A NURSING HOME RESIDENT?

## Who, Me? A Nursing Home Resident?

A nursing home resident?

Me? Yes, me! And my spouse — both of us healthy, employed homeowners from Oregon. What were we doing as patients in an Indiana long-term-care facility — eating with residents, attending therapy and activity sessions, occupying a room by the nursing station?

Fiction? Or was I fantasizing?

No, it really happened. I had just presented a seminar for the staff of the Byron Health Center in Fort Wayne when boldly I asked the administrator: "May we possibly stay on a while, Mr. Katsanis?* May we take this chance to view the world as patients — may we experience the reality of life in a nursing home?"

Graciously consenting, Mr. Katsanis did me one better. "Spend a few days with us," he offered. "Take five. Roam about at will. Observe staff, residents, volunteers, families of patients. Become a part of our big, happy family."

---

*His *real* name, used with permission.

I'd heard that "big happy family" spiel before! And I wondered if here they could justify this claim. Thus began a memorable week, a highlight of my career.

Plainly, no institution, especially a 500-bed one, can mask its true image, "put on the dog" for five days straight, just to impress visitors. And so, what we would observe would be the normal daily routine of this non-profit facility. No events staged, no special favors for one who would "eagle-eye" every nook and cranny; one who might just pick up her pen and publicize irregularities or critique the experience. However, Mr. Katsanis is not worried.

My spouse and I settle in. Residents accept us as one of them, unaware of our status here. When our time is up, we will have experienced life in an unusual, and a really "good" facility which, we will discover, has earned the right to stand tall as a national model for long term care.

Wednesday, our first full day, the administrator takes the time to orient us. We tour the place. We meet staff and clients. Mr. Katsanis has a flair for remembering names. To every resident we meet in the halls he gives a personal greeting. He knows their interests and accomplishments. Many embrace him with affection, returning the love which he radiates. "Sometimes I slip up on names," he admits, "especially of the new residents." However, not once do we catch him groping for a name. Says my husband: "What greater compliment can an administrator pay to his guests?"

No wonder residents beam at the mention of his name. "Our Tom — he's the greatest!" they brag or, "Mrs. Katsanis and the four children really care for us!" Several residents remarked: "If I *must* live away from home, this is the place I'm happiest to be!"

After the tour, the administrator shows us films. As in many Care Centers, there is no end to the handwork on display. Lovely shots of hooked rugs, horticultural exhibits, individual garden plots, knitted items. But the film which most intrigued us was the one showing three elders in wheelchairs placed in the basket of a huge balloon. They are lifted up seventy-five feet, airborne for a spectacular view of the surrounding area. "For $200.00 we rent this balloon," explains Mr. Katsanis, "an annual event during our summer picnic. They love it!" To which I could only murmur: "Darned if *I'd* be brave enough to lift off in that thing!"

Originating as the old County Poor Farm, the Byron Health Center was once a remote, dismal "cage" for the ill and indigent. Inmates clawed at iron bars, hoping to escape. But thirty years ago, despite public scepticism, Tom Katsanis took charge and ordered: "Remove all bars." His philosophy? "Regardless of a client's physical or mental status, staff must uphold the dignity of each person who lives here."

We like what we read on a brass plaque over the front portal. "The goal for every client is rehabilitation so that, whenever possible, that person may be returned to hearth and home." No mere platitude, this goal is often met. Last month, seventeen residents returned to the larger community. If in the old days inmates yearned to escape this morbid poor farm, today long lines of prospective clients await without trepidation their turn to be admitted.

Before elaborating on life in this health center, I ask myself just what, exactly, is it here that contributes to the overall aura of contentment. How does the staff attain such intangibles for the residents as "meaningful living," or "mental and spiritual growth?" What, precisely, is their formula for "quality care?"

On our second day of residency, we begin to find answers. At breakfast we note some ambulatory clients proudly displaying lapel badges: *"I am a Resident Volunteer"* and as the day wears on, we see these people circulating, pushing wheelchairs, feeding the helpless, delivering mail, caring for goldfish, watering plants, gainfully employed in the library and gift shops. Wherever possible, residents have the chance to serve and use their time and skills. And this, I believe, is the secret. A sense of joy permeating the place. *Administration recognizes the human need to be needed and appreciated.* And so, residents as well as community volunteers join hands to enrich the lives of one another.

As for those ubiquitous community volunteers, the place is a buzz of activity, much like what I saw in Chinese old age homes. It is said: "An institution must not be a one-way, or dead-end street. *There is no such thing as a good nursing home which does not invite support from the larger community."* At the Byron Health Center, this support is powerful.

That afternoon we attend a music therapy session. In the soundproof room, a group is enjoying the Schubert "Unfinished Symphony." At intervals, the therapist, with her M.S. degree from Purdue, comments or invites discussion. Members of the group had once been music lovers, instrumentalists or teachers of classical music. Emotionally and intellectually they drink in the great sounds, lost in the ecstacy of the moment.

Walking down the hall we see a sign: "Dentist." Dr. Jones asks us to come in. At the moment, an 89-year-old woman is being fitted for new lowers. Here a belief prevails that a person is *never too old to be comfortable* and that good dental care contributes to enjoyment of foods, good nutrition and better appearance, all leading to enhanced self-esteem.

The same with eyeglasses and hearing aids. These are kept current — essential if one is to keep up with reading, crafts and lifelong learning. We meet the optician who is making one of his tri-weekly visits. Because many clients have sensory impairment, it is good that within the total care plan these needs for adjustment are fulfilled. A newly-admitted man whose glasses had not been adjusted in 15 years was brought in for an eye examination. With new glasses he was able to resume woodcarving, a hobby he had abandoned. His morale thrives.

In his office, the podiatrist is giving foot care to a diabetic patient. He, too, functions importantly within the facility. "Those that can walk," he says, "let them walk for as long as possible." All deserve and get the best of care for again, "nobody is too old to be comfortable." All services, including medical care, are packaged in the reasonable monthly charge — one which compares favorably with facilities which provide many services at extra cost. A person's ability to pay is not always the criterion for admission. Human needs supercede all other considerations.

Now it is Friday, our third day as residents. We are invited to attend a Care Plan session. As always, Mr. Katsanis presides. Having worked in nine nursing homes in five states, I can truly say that this session is extraordinary. Never have I seen such efficient use of time. Five days a week at 9 a.m. sharp, the Administrator calls the meeting to order. Exactly thirty minutes later it is adjourned. Meanwhile, there is a whirl of activity. Each session assesses the progress of three designated patients. Department heads attend the session, as does the resident chaplain, resident physician, activities director, therapists, dietician, and social worker. Often the patient who is under consideration attends and sometimes his family. This improves overall awareness of the status and goals for that resident. Families cooperate with staff, knowing that they function importantly in contributing to the well-being of their loved one and to the home. During the session, each professional is called upon to make suggestions. Constructive comments fill the air such as: "Can we meet our goal of sending Mrs. Cassidy home this week?" or, "Mrs. Hansen seems more outgoing since she has worked in occupational therapy projects. How else can we help her?"

Time now for food talk. Imagine if you can the challenge of feeding 500 residents plus a staff of 400, three times a day! Rather difficult to achieve the ideal of "gracious dining!" There is still improvement to be made for it is not easy to silence altogether the clattering of dishes from the kitchen area or to provide a fresh flower for each table. We miss the soft background music which so greatly enhances relaxation to the diners. But we like the Center's idea of cafeteria-style service, which not only gives ambulatory residents on regular diets their freedom of choice, but provides choice for many diabetic patients as well. Sugarless foods with their colored markers are easy to spot and those on restricted diets live up to the trust placed in them that they will not "snitch" forbidden fruit. We enjoyed walking down the line and serving ourselves. Far more dignified than plunking a pre-filled tray before a client with the unspoken implication: "Here, eat. Like it or lump it!"

The food is good. We find variety and color for taste and eye appeal. As we eat, rather than the usual silence found in most institutions, we note animated chatter among residents. Care is also placed in the skilled care units that the meals are attractive, unhurriedly served, with emphasis on enjoyment.

My spouse and I scan the bulletin board for Friday's activities. We settle for the Poetry class. Says the therapist: "Poetry draws people out of their shells; unearths the rough spots of guilt and hostility; stimulates the emotions and intellect. Like music, it calms the restless mind." We note that when a group gathers to share a poem and reactions to that poem, a bond is forged. We rejoice that this therapist likes those silly verses from the "Golden Trashery of Ogden Nashery," which encourage laughter. Before our very eyes we see stress dissolving as we all hoot over the limerick:

> A clergyman out in Dumont
> Keeps a tropical fish in his font.
> Though it always surprises
> The babes he baptises
> It seems to be just what they want!

Already it is Saturday. After socializing with a few sun-worshippers outside, we dress up to attend a gala celebration in honor of eight newly admitted residents. Lovely decorations and snacks, a lively resident band, wide smiles on every face, spirited singing and clapping all add to the merriment. How they all joined in with "Happy Days are Here Again," and "Glory Halleluia," and "Bicycle Built for Two!"

Here comes Mr. Katsanis, who never misses these welcoming festivities. Pointing us out to the group, he asks my spouse and me to "say a word" over the microphone. We say a word all right! We express our pleasure in sharing their lives in this home-away-from-home; our joy in sensing the spirit of cameraderie; our realization that here it is not just an empty claim on a public relations brochure, but it is literally so that this is one Big Happy Family!

As the party ends a Mr. White wheels himself over to us and grumps: "Happy family? My foot! I wish I were home!" We see how deeply he misses his family, but it is wholesome that he feels free to express his thoughts. Relaying the message to the chaplain, I hope that Mr. White might soon show progress in his rehabilitation and soon consider himself a part of the group. He's been here only a week. Some others who at first felt the same way now make a positive contribution to the home, often helped in so doing by the Resident Volunteer Corps.

That overall aura of contentment stems in part from the Resident Council, one of the strongest in the U.S. Recently this group flew its president, wheelchair and all, to Washington D.C. to meet with other nursing home council representatives. Each month this Indiana group publishes a newsletter. Thus, residents enjoy democratic "say" in the affairs of the home. Should a complaint be voiced, the council either settles it or posts it on the bulletin board outside the office of the Administrator. Checking the board daily, Mr. Katsanis respects the rights of the complainer to be heard, works with that person to iron out the difficulty. He never leaves a problem dangling in mid-air.

Sunday — our final day. First we attend Protestant service, then Catholic mass. The chapel overflows with worshippers. Staff takes pains to bring in even the most disabled patients, thus preserving their sense of belonging. Mr. Katsanis knows the value of fulfilling spititual needs along with needs of mind and body: the Sabbath is observed by Jewish residents. Later he takes us with his family to Fort Wayne for a fine dinner.

One more observation. The Byron Health Center staff understands the value of touch. During our visit we have seen much nonverbal communication — touching, backrubs, etc. It is contagious for now, Sunday evening, as the hour approaches for us to fly back to Oregon, we find ourselves bear-hugging members of the staff, the administrator (he's "Tom" to us now) and residents.

Parting is not easy. How shall I ever forget the warm embrace of Marie, that fragile little lady? Hugging her I feared I might break every bone in her body!

Gathering around, residents shower us with snapshots and handmade gifts. One woman presents us with her original poem, dedicated to "Our Tom and His Family." And Greg, that handsome, bearded old gentleman presses into my husband's hand a piece of gingerbread to enjoy on the flight home.

Yes, it's hard to pull away. We've so enjoyed new friendships with those who, as Pearl Buck described them, "have come a little farther in the experience of life." We assure staff and residents that we will always retain joyous memories of this very special place.

As we board the plane, I know that I must share this experience with readers, and that I will urge them: "If ever you get the chance, take up temporary residency, incognito, in a quality nursing home. Eat, sleep, play, enter fully into the life of these beautiful people. For here, if anywhere, the phrase 'quality care' takes on meaning. I guarantee you an enriching experience."

Who, me? A nursing home patient? Fact indeed, not fiction. As our plane becomes airborne we sense an awareness that for most people, even the institutionalized, late life need not mean stagnation. It can be a time of continuing growth, living and loving. And it can be that *only* if people have something to live for.

We ponder more deeply our own futures. During the sunset of

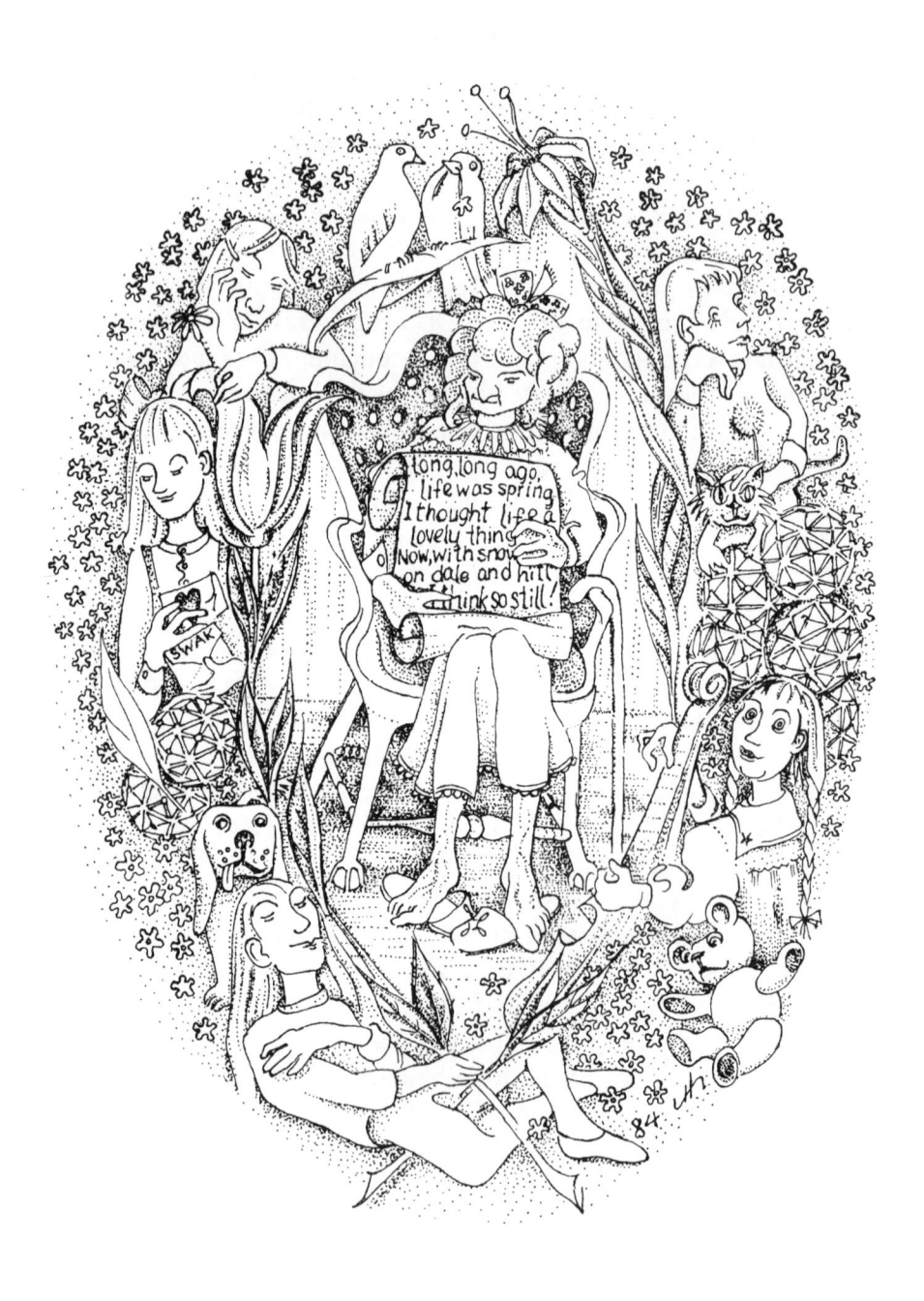

Long, long ago,
life was spring
I thought life a
lovely thing
Now, with snow
on dale and hill
I think so still!

*our* lives, will we embrace the simple philosophy of the Byron Health Center, that *life is for the living?* That life to the very end should be savored? That for the bedridden as well as for the ambulatory person, we can open up the paths for purposeful lives? Will our own outlook be as upbeat as that of one little woman who tapped my arm to share a verse she had memorized?

LONG, LONG AGO, WHEN LIFE WAS SPRING
I THOUGHT LIFE WAS A LOVELY THING:
AND NOW, WITH SNOW ON DALE AND HILL
I THINK SO STILL!

*For the institutionalized, how
important are links to the past?*

## CHAPTER SEVEN

## PERSONAL POSSESSIONS:
### Trash or Treasure?

## Personal Possessions:
## Trash or Treasure?*

"It's unsanitary. Throw it out!"

So insisted the nursing staff, the housekeeping staff and the inspectors.

"Yes, it's got to go. That handbag of Tillie's — it must be fifty years old. Motheaten. A disgrace. Get rid of it!"

But how? At the very mention, 94-year-old Tillie would rage, stamp her feet. And at night, twisting the strap around her wrist, she clasped the bag to her bosom as she slept.

"Batty old battleaxe!" muttered someone. "Why there isn't even anything *in* the bag!"

Rather a problem. For you see, this nursing home had a reputation to maintain. Spotless, shining, immaculate. What if a visitor noticed that eyesore?

Embarrassing!

A showdown was inevitable. One night as Tillie dozed, an employee crept into her room, eased the strap from its mooring and tiptoed back to the lighted hall. Sighs of relief from the staff.

*Originally published in " Geriatric Care", June, 1984
(Eymann Publications, Box 3577, Reno, NV 89505

Sure enough, upon opening the bag, they found nothing inside. Nothing, that is, except a tattered blue handkerchief, a cheap dime-store ring, a snapshot, faded beyond recognition. "Well, that's that," said the employee as she tossed the thing into the trashcan. We'll just get her a new one."

At six the next morning, Tillie discovered her loss. In disbelief she tossed her covers aside, scrambled about ever more frantically, then the wailing began. Setting up a howl one could hear down the hall, for days she carried on ceaselessly. Everyone tried but nobody could console her. She pounded, kicked, cursed and tossed aside the new handbag. Not a single employee saw the need to sit with Tillie and hear her out. Instead, a sedative was ordered.

It was at this time that I was hired by this facility for night duty. All talk still focused on Tillie. The air reeked with a dozen versions of what had triggered Tillie's "senile" behavior. Taking the direct route, I decided to ask her personally how she felt and why.

At midnight I entered her cubicle. She was awake. Reflected in the light from the hall, tears glistened on her wrinkled cheeks.

"Tell me about your handbag, Tillie," I said. "Why do you take this so hard?"

"It's not so much the bag itself," she moaned. "The staff here is real kind. They got me a new one. It was what was *in* the bag." I reached for her hand. It was trembling.

"But I heard there was nothing in it — just some knick-knacks of no value."

"That's right, Nancy — of no value to them others. But you know that old hankie? I kept it all these years. It was a present from my mother — 'something blue' to wear at my wedding."

"And what of the ring, Tillie? Couldn't I get you another one, maybe even more pretty and shiney?"

"That ring? Back in 1912 when we was wed, my Jake was just a farmhand. He wanted a ring on my finger. For twenty-five cents he bought it. I can hear him now, the way he said: 'Tillie, Sweetheart, when I'm rich I'll buy you a real ring.' Later he did get me a nice fancy one, but that first one — that was my keepsake, my token of our vow. Jake was my love, my one and only love. I never married again."

"And the snapshot, Tillie?"

Now she was sobbing. "With the ring, that snapshot was all I

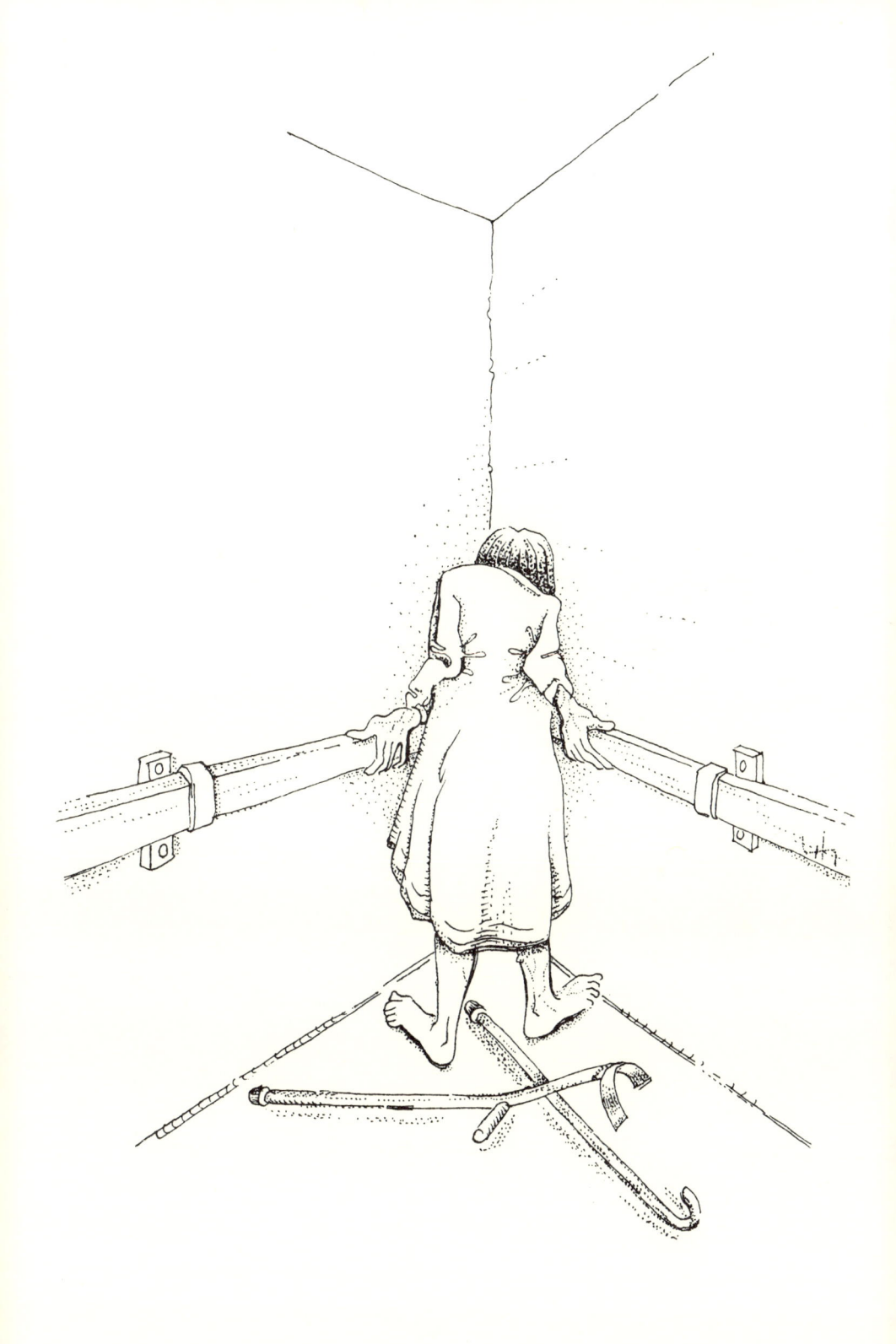

had left of Jake. I lost him during the 1918 flu epidemic. Years later our little house burned to the ground. Everything was lost — scrapbooks, furniture, everything. But I saved the handbag. And in it were the hankie, the snapshot and the ring."

I put my arms around Tillie. What could I say?

*Aftermath of Stroke:*
*Triumph or Tragedy?*
*My eyewitness account.*

## CHAPTER EIGHT

# THE SHUSH-UP OF MRS. PARK

# The Shush-Up of Mrs. Park

Such excitement! Today Mrs. Amy Park goes home. Her "doctoring days" in the long term care wing are over.

Felled one year ago by a devastating stroke (cerebrovascular accident), paralyzed and aphasic, it seemed she was beyond hope. But now, because somebody cared and took the initiative, she has made an astonishing comeback.

With tears of gratitude, Mrs. Park slips a note into the pocket of her favorite nurse, Ruth Hall. Borrowing from a poem, she wrote:

    Bless you, Ruth, for what you have made of me;
    Bless you for passing over all the foolish things in me
    And for drawing out what no one else
    Had looked quite far enough to find.
    Bless you, Ruth, for making out of my life
    Not a reproach, but a song.

Now, Mrs. Park herself will tell her story.

### The Call to Action

"Ruth is a jewel," she begins. "I'll never forget her. Not discouraged by my dismal prognosis, she went ahead, gently exercising my weak limbs, helping me to form words and sentences. An aura of calm surrounded Ruth. When she said: 'Mrs. Park, you will walk again' I believed her and was motivated to work towards this goal.

"That incredible nurse! She opened up every path to me that had seemed forever closed. To her the word 'chronic' did not mean 'hopeless.' Instead, it was her trumpet call. Her question was not *whether* to strike back at stroke, but *how* to convince others that, even with me, this could be done.

"One day in the hall I overheard the head nurse saying: 'Ruth, I do not share your optimism for Amy Park — you know what Dr. Morton said.' Complete silence. Then, 'Why do you overly encourage her, Ruth? At her age, it's not worth it!'

"My heart turned a somersault. But when Ruth reentered my room her expression restored my hopes. Evidently I *was* worth it!

"To Ruth, I was worth the time it took to help me into my lovely nightgown, not as simple to don as one of those slit-back monstrosities that make you feel like an inmate. Makeup, too, and always an attractive hairdo. One afternoon when she exclaimed: 'Oh, Mrs. Park, you look so glamorous! You should be Queen-of-the-May!' I almost burst my buttons. Because Ruth had recognized my inner needs, I was able to accept with good grace the rigors of rehabilitation.

### Time for Teamwork

"As my improvement became evident, other staff members pitched in, taking credit for the change. Finally Dr. Morton ordered a complete therapy program — physical, speech, occupational — the whole works! Now everyone believed in me. I *will* get better. I *will* go home, someday!

### Homeward Bound

"As Jim, my husband, escorts me from the long term care wing, I'm grinning like a Cheshire cat. They're all waving goodbye. In the excitement as I hug Ruth, my cane is knocked over. Words stick in my throat. Someday I'll be able to tell her what it meant to have a nurse who looked behind the illness to the real me. Never pushing, yet always dangling before my eyes a rainbow. Oh how I treasured her manner — the way she looked at and touched me; the tone of her voice. I could always sense her loving concern. Tears cloud my eyes — tears of affection for a nurse who cared.

"We're off! Goodbye! Goodbye, everyone! Goodbye!

"Our little Chevy rounds the bend on Maple Street. There's our house! Oh, and here comes old Joey-Jowls, our St. Bernard dog, lumbering over the lawn to greet his master. Suddenly he spies *me*! Letting out a colossal howl, his great body shudders with excitement.

"Neighbors gather around. For a moment I am overwhelmed — transported into an unreal world. Jim steadies my arm. Now I know I am really home.

### Fanning Frustrations

"It's our first evening together. As soft music fills the room, I unwind from the whirl of the day and begin to reminisce. Jim and Joey-Jowls are such good listeners!

"Remember Dear," I began, "how rough it was at first? Even though Ruth steadied the ship, oh those frustrations — the limb that wouldn't work, the speech that sounded like a mouthful of hot mush. I didn't even know the word 'aphasia' existed. Remember how I used to bawl at the drop of a hat? Jim, you were so embarrassed! But Ruth to the rescue. How her eyes danced as she said: 'Guess what, Mrs. Park — starting today, you're in a *new phase* of your recovery. The crying spells are past history — they are over.'

"How did she *know*? Anyway, I did quit it and a new phase was launched. Say, Jim, come to think of it, do you suppose Ruth *invented* that "phase" bit?

"And oh, the time I deliberately crashed my dinner tray to the floor. Stew, gravy, potatoes flying every which way; wobbly red jello oozing from the night-stand! Was I ever obnoxious! But no sermon from Ruth. Jim, I never told you this part, but the next day, so help me, I did the very same thing again, only this time the soup splashed as far off as the window pane. For a second Ruth looked at me. I bet she was wild inside! Then it came. 'Mrs. Park,' she said, 'for your information it so happens that only yesterday I was reading the carpet manufacturer's pamphlet on '"Proper Care of Commercial Carpets" and he recommends — and I quote: 'To insure long wear and brilliant lustre, douse carpet frequently and thoroughly with meatballs, gravy, pea soup and tossed salad.'

"I began to titter. The knotted nerves loosened. Now my laughter became uproarious. My wheelchair shook. Joining in, Ruth put her arms around me and together we enjoyed the absurdity. Of course this ended my food-flipping phase but better still, she had helped me to maintain my self-esteem and cope with frustrations. If only more staff could appreciate the value of the light touch! She knew when I needed a reassuring hug or a gentle backrub to iron out the kinks of anxiety.

"Ruth saw me, not as just the 'case' in Room 76, but as a whole person. To her I was Mrs. Amy Park, dog lover, gardener, church member, poet, homemaker — a human being with feelings, memories, opinions. One who longed for respect and independence. Total care for the total me. Yet when I praised her, the simple response was: 'I do only what any caring nurse would do.' to Ruth, I was not an 'it' to be manipulated, but a 'thou' to be honored.

### Between Triumph and Tragedy

"It's been a happy week at home. Jim is an angel the way he's adjusted to my slower pace.

'Isn't it time to spread our wings again, dear?' he asked. 'It's Sunday. Let's go back to church.' My momentary enthusiasm fell flat as I recalled those six steps up front. (We were not aware that a ramp had been installed.) And so, instead, we took a drive. But oh, how I whacked my head on the low ceiling of the car! Haven't auto designers ever heard of the handicapped or the elderly?

"On Monday, another disappointment. 'Lassie' was showing at the Paramount, but wouldn't I trip over legs in those cramped row seats? We stayed home. Everywhere — at the bank, at certain stores we kept discovering barriers. Heavy doors, escalators, crowded elevators which scare me to death.

"Came Saturday, the day of the Little League championship game, Colby and Jenny, our grand-nephew and niece, would shine. We promised we'd attend. But what about those steep bleachers? And I couldn't sit *outside* the field to get clobbered, as Jim warned me, by a foul ball. Foiled again, we stayed home.

"By now I was churning. This week had been a fiasco. I'd heard of this "youth-oriented" society, but now, for the first time, I see oldsters like us as excess baggage. Even my home-health nurse would warn me, sometimes, about the barriers out there. 'It's better than it was ten years ago,' she'd say, 'but our town is dragging its feet.'

" 'Jim,' I peeved, 'where *can* I go? In our neighborhood even sidewalks are lacking. I want to get out and do things. Have I got the Black Plague, or is Mayville subtly telling me: 'Get lost, you old has-been!'

"Rehabilitated? Rehabilitated *for what*? I wept. Is it for me to sit all day at home, squeezed out of the human race? Is it for me to backslide, to get depressed and housebound like old Mr. Jarvis next door? After all my rehabilitation efforts? Can't the home-health people fit me into their schedule more often? There are so many other people with priority over me. Jim, we've got to live a little while we still have time. Does anybody care? Doesn't *anybody*? I'm so tired. Help me to bed, Dear. Guess I don't feel my best today."

### Transition

Two months later, Jim suffered a heart attack. Amy was inconsolable. She found him dead, slumped on the porch floor.

The weeks passed. As her nieces and nephews got caught up in the hubbub of Christmas, their visits dwindled. Maddened by loneliness, Amy hardly touched her food brought in by the Meals-on-Wheels people. No one to sit with her. To eat alone? Unbearable. Most of her food she scraped into the dog dish. And always by her side her devoted Joey-Jowls would raise his sad brown eyes as if to say: "But you've still got *me*!"

### Tragedy

Winter closed in. The snows fell. Harsh winds rattled Amy's window panes. The ambulance came, taking her to the hospital. Pneumonia. Ruth visited, only to be shocked by the gaunt look on Amy's face.

And then, after alternative housing had been explored and rejected, the inevitable happened. Amy's nieces placed her in a nursing home, 70 miles from Mayville. By New Year's Day, Amy's home was up for sale, her furniture auctioned off. But the final numbing blow — her adored Joey-Jowls was sent to the pound.

Amy's world collapsed. The same Mrs. Park who, five months earlier had jubilantly returned home is now widowed, uprooted, her life surrendered to strangers. Although nieces come occasionally to visit, their superficial chitchat does nothing to divert her from deep despondency.

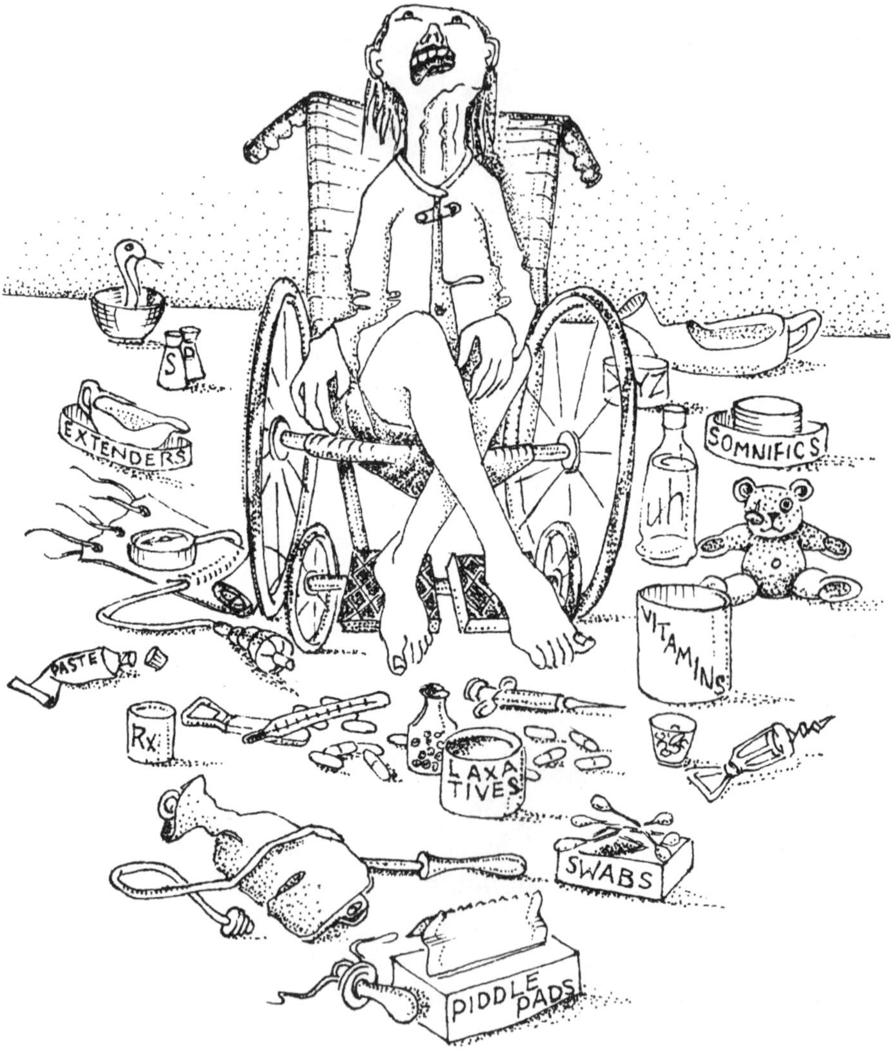

EXTENDERS
SOMNIFICS
VITAMINS
PASTE
Rx
LAXA TIVES
SWABS
PIDDLE PADS

## The Sunset Nursing Home

Like an arid desert, the days stretch before her. Amy feels useless. Busy aides wheel rather than walk her to the bathroom — it's quicker and easier. She is losing strength, losing independence.

The Sunset Home is immaculate. In the spacious Visitors' Lounge, one finds lush gold carpeting, colorful paintings, oversize imitation plants — all the latest decor. The administrator is proud to show off the lounge — he almost struts. The public is impressed. On the grand piano sits a massive fan-shaped gladiola 'floral arrangement' — a leftover from the GRIMES MORTUARY. (Mr. Grimes frequently unloads these vulgarities on the Sunset Home. And because staff chooses to believe that "residents don't know the difference," nobody bothers to rearrange the flowers in individual vases.)

Of course, Sunset is certified by the State Health Department. "One of the state's finest facilities," according to inspectors. But to the visitor, the "elegant" atmosphere is misleading. How can one be expected to sense the intangible — the great inherent flaw of Sunset, that is, a lopsided emphasis on human values? Here, emphasis is placed on expert physical care. In this the staff excels. But staff bypasses most of the available professional workshops which focus on the physical, yes, but stressing equally the spiritual, emotional, intellectual needs of aging persons. Staff professes but rarely practices the art of "total care."

Inexperienced young nurses and aides, incapable of conversing with their clients, view them as objects on which to perform procedures. Aides are hired willy-nilly with little regard for their competence or for their motives in applying for the job. Disgruntled, they rush through the day's routine, complaining about their supervisors, the workload and the pay. While insisting that "our budget does not allow for more employees," the administrator accepts as inevitable that "hiring-firing-quitting" marathon. Residents are bewildered by the whirling kaleidoscope of unfamiliar faces.

Although special diets are provided, the dietitian in this home, unlike some in that profession, hardly knows a face — just the client name cards on trays. There is a lovely sunny dining room but many, like Amy, pick at their food in the solitude of their own "cells." A dress protector is tied around her neck, only they call it a "bib." Her dessert is snitched by an aide who can't afford to buy a lunch — that takes too large a chunk out of her insultingly small paycheck.

Occasionally a minister drops in on Amy. (She wonders why nobody ever asked permission to use her first name.) Unable to establish a meaningful relationship with her, he hides behind a Scripture reading then hastily departs. A priest mumbles something unintelligible, which the hard-of-hearing miss entirely, rushes a ritual, and he, too, vanishes into thin air. The Jewish residents, with their Rabbi, seem to fare better.

### Regression

Mrs. Park is regressing. By now she is being lifted in and out of bed. Outside her window she sees the snow-covered trees. Only a few winter birds are braving the cold. "Staff never took me out in good weather," she weeps. "I miss my garden." Then, in anguish she cries: "Oh, Jim, why did you have to leave me?"

Nurse Ruth knew well that despair leads to apathy; apathy leads inactivity; inactivity leads to loss of function. At an alarming rate, Mrs. Park is losing physical and mental function.

Church groups come to sing "at" rather than *with* the residents. Girl Scouts bring cookies, rather than the ingredients so that they may work together, creating, enjoying togetherness. One look at Amy shows the ravages of isolation, the lack of meaningful participation, the loss of self-respect. Reduced to a "roleless role" her life is being merely sustained, not enriched. After a recent visit, Ruth found it intolerable to see those eyes, now without expression. Amy, rapidly aging, has given up.

Mrs. Park is the latest to join that faceless throng of the catheterized, chronically ill aged — a burden to herself, a burden to others. Nurses and aides who have not helped her to maintain bodily function refer to her, in her presence, as a "difficult case." Words such as "diapers," "potty-chair" and bib jar her nerves — words she had thought applied only to infants. Unfamiliar treatments are pushed on her without prior explanation. Her body has been confiscated. It lies exposed while aides go for linens. Hurriedly washed and dressed, she feels like trash. Retreating ever further into a world of her own, Amy becomes increasingly overwhelmed. She can no longer cope.

Now, 3:00 a.m., after hours of restless tossing, she yearns for the balm of sleep. Her thoughts drift back to the turn of the century when they advertised "Asylums for the Needy," "Homes for Incurables," and yes, even "Shelters for the Doomed." Lights flicker on her wall as bare branches sway over the outdoor neon sign which reads: "SUNSET HEALTH CARE FACILITY." A feeling of guilt overcomes her as in her mind an outrageous thought takes shape. "Shouldn't that sign be reworded? Shouldn't it read: 'SUNSET SHELTER FOR THE DOOMED?' "

### Chain Reaction

Sunset's house physician, Dr. Wilcox, has been learning more and more about stroke, less and less about Amy Park. Only once has he seen her face to face. Ambitious, always eager to see dramatic hospital cases and cures, he views her as hopeless. Lacking training in both the biological and psycho-social aspects of aging, his stock reply to most problems is: What can you expect — it's your age!" — as he rushes on to complete his gang visits.

The attitude of Dr. Wilcox rubs off on the staff which comes to believe that Amy is neither clinically nor socially worthy of a doctor's time. Craving attention, Amy begins to shake her bed rails. Repeatedly scolded, she is told to "quit it and shut up." Now desperate, she resorts to the continuous ringing of her call bell, whereupon an exasperated aide, inflicting a sharp slap on her buttocks, moves the bell out of reach. Her life-line now pulled, Amy experiences in her abdomen a weird, sinking sensation. Clutching the air, pleading, moaning, she is taken to the farthest end of the hall where she will be less of a disturbance. Contacted by phone, Dr. Wilcox suggests restraints and extra sedation, together with the comment: "That woman belongs in the nuthouse!" This remark, becoming a classic among the staff, is kicked around like a football from old to new employees; a stigma for the duration of Amy's life.

The disease of "helplessness" is taking its toll. As though she were a zombie, the staff speaks of Amy in her presence. "She'll be dead in a month," quips a pert little nurse as with professional precision she makes a wrinkle-free bed. Raising her head with a jerk, Amy's look of panic goes unnoticed.

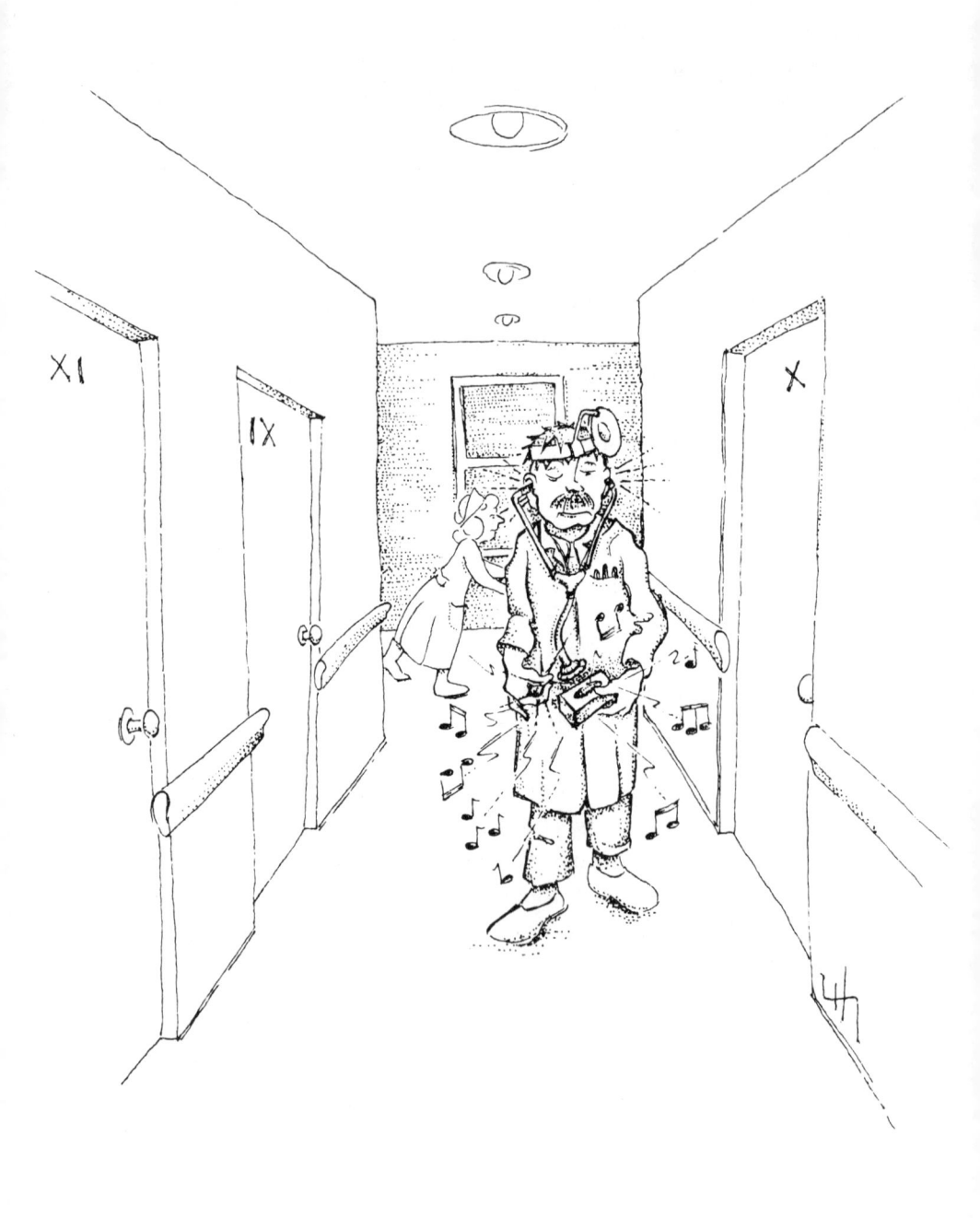

That nurse could be right. Sitting mute in her wheelchair, heavily drugged, Amy's will to live has been smothered.

It was just three weeks later that Ruth noticed in the obituary column:

Mrs. Amy Park
Sunset Nursing Home
... of natural causes
GRIMES MORTUARY IN CHARGE

Telephoning Sunset, Ruth heard a hurried voice: "Amy? Amy Park? Oh, yes, no known cause of death — just old age. Dr. Wilcox says she's better off now." As she slowly lowered the receiver, Ruth heard the voice continuing: "By the way, Miss Hall, next Tuesday we are having a ribbon-cutting ceremony to celebrate our new 50-bed wing. Do hope you can attend."

Ruth knows that loss of control over one's life can tip the scales towards death. She fears for her other patients as she reads the words of psychologist Martin Seligman: "Depression is the belief in one's own helplessness. This can bring on unexpected death. The rejected, the handicapped and the old have all been victims."

Mrs. Park is dead. But still today, within the walls of Sunset, there continues to rage, unchecked, that very epidemic which claimed her life. One by one, patients who have not received orders for therapy or rehabilitation are succumbing to this insidious malady, "helplessness," as it takes its lethal toll. Wring out the old? Yes, like a washcloth, in many areas of the U.S. we are wringing out our elders, snuffing out their potential for a meaningful late-life experience.

At the Sunset Home, no room will remain vacant for more than a day. To ring in the new, there is always that waiting list of about 90 persons. And while the voice of authority proudly chants: "In this institution we give the finest care," the chorus swells to a mightly crescendo: "Yes, the state rates us second to none. Imagine, *not one single bedsore in the entire place!*"

## Post Script

After the funeral, Amy was laid to rest beside her husband, Jim. Ruth attended the service. So did the two nieces who, because of "other commitments," had seen very little of Amy during the past year.

When they returned to pick up Amy's belongings, the next-of-kin was satisfied when told that "everything possible was done to prevent bedsores," and that "your Aunt Amy was kept pleasantly occupied and happy with her many friends here at Sunset." The nieces were also reassured to hear the stock phrase: "She passed away peacefully in her sleep."

It was also gratifiying for them to see as they passed through the lounge their costly, massive, fan-shaped gladiola "floral arrangement" perched up there on the grand piano.

Truly spectacular!

*Should Americans retire, simply to sit snug in a state of sexless senility?*

## CHAPTER NINE

## SEXUALITY AT *ANY* AGE:
## Part of Being Human

## Sexuality at Any Age: Part of Being Human

There she goes, that voluptuous blonde,
swinging her hips as she sashays down the street.
And there he sits, the 90-year old, perched by his rest-home
window, binoculars in hot pursuit!

Absurd — this ageless interest in the opposite sex? Not in Equador, Pakistan or in the Soviet Caucasus. Surveys by Dr. Alexander Leaf, Massachusetts General Hospital, show that in those countries, centennarians work hard, live at home, enjoy respect *and* remain sexually active. But most American hospitals and nursing homes scorn this concept. Countless handicapped and/or elderly people find their love needs ignored by the institution, shoved under the rug by relatives. Come, let's confront this.

Consider that prize cliché: "We *all* need love." Why does it so often exclude long-lived persons?

From birth to retirement, most Americans cling to family and friends. But in that last cycle of life, when a sense of love and belonging is more crucially needed than ever, comes a shattering blow. Rarely are total love needs recognized. In fact, should an aged patriarch or matriarch even *hint* they've *heard* of sex — quick, the tranquilizer!

From cradle to casket, however, love dominates our thoughts. As the vine needs sunlight, so do people of all ages need nurturing. Withhold this and tension mounts. Like bread from a toaster, up pops bizarre behavior or complaints, real or imagined.

Claiming that "here all their love needs are taken care of," health-care facilities, particularly nursing homes, justify this myth to the tune of millions of dollars a year in sedatives. Society accepts as normal that galaxy of strange noises, odors, glassy eyes, drooling mouths, slumped bodies. *Wake up, America!* The quick fix, sedation, may not be the solution - may not be what your loved one needs.

| 5 | SELF |
|---|---|
|   | (actualization, to create, explore) |
| 4 | ESTEEM |
|   | (Value of self) |
| 3 | LOVE NEEDS |
|   | (To love and be loved) |
| 2 | SAFETY |
|   | (To feel secure) |
| 1 | PHYSIOLOGICAL |
|   | (Food, water, etc.) |

**Maslow's Hierarchy of Needs**

In this chart, love needs follow closely on the heels of basic food and safety requirements. *Not one* of these five essentials can we tag with an expiration date.

Despite current gerontic research which finds that sexual interest and ability can last into late life, many institutions assume that elders are content to sit snug in a state of sexless senility. Our "enlightened" society notwithstanding, we must ask some hard questions:

*What is the outlook for the aging person who maintains interest in the opposite sex?*

*By what right, in somber moral tones, do we censor the private affairs of any couple, any age?*

*On whose authority do we limit them to "kidstuff" handholding?*

*When, oh when will society put adequate emphasis on the total psychosocial needs of older persons?*

*Where in the Bible does it say: "At age sixty-five, thy love life shall lapse?"\**

---

\*Read what the Bible tells of Abram and Hager who had their son Ishmael when Abram was 86 years old (Genesis 17:1-19). The account goes on with the Almighty God changing Abram's name to Abraham, and the name of his barren wife to Sarah, and that they have their son Isaac when he is 100 and she is 90 years old. Thus, it appears, the Almighty endorses sexiness in the elderly.

## Would You Do It Differently?

Gert, the nursing aide, enters Room 30. She finds Ralph locked in the arms of Mae, his wife. Gert splits. It had long been evident how sorely he missed their marital intimacy, for his roving eye penetrated any female contour he encountered. Nurses avoided him like a viper. *Patients' Rights* notwithstanding, privacy here is a rare commodity. And so today, overcome with "oomph," Ralph makes a beeline for the bed of his beloved. Alas, he cannot lock the door!

Without knocking, Gert enters. Gert exits, jet-propelled. Outside the couple's room she pins me to the wall, tells me her problem. (And it *is her* problem!) I tell her: "Shut the door tightly, post a 'DO NOT DISTURB' sign."

All their married life, Ralph and Mae have shared a bed. But have you ever seen a double bed in a nursing home?

For centuries the female of our species has been repressed. Only the "shady-lady-in-red" was credited with having any sexual nature at all. (You've come a long way, Baby!) Today it is known that, barring certain health conditions, the libido lasts a lifetime. The American male, despite a gradual decline, can sustain desire and performance into and beyond the 90s, according to his self esteem and expectations. Yet prudish attitudes persist, rubbing off from one person to another, as on that day when Nurse Carol gunned down George and Minnie, the inseparables. Anna, the aide, was witness.

## Substituting Sedation for Sex

The pair, quiet and content, is watching TV. But today, so very tenderly, their eyes meet, his head tilts towards hers, his hand finds her knee. Just then Carol glances up from her desk. She opens fire. "Anna, get those two apart. What will people think!" But something was ignored. Over the years, George and Minnie had endured the loss of loved ones, countless tearful separations. Now they were dealt another heartwrench. Of course there's always sedation. *Better blah than blissful*! Stuff them into a convenient assexual vacuum! But can sedation substitute for full living? Strange therapy for feelings of isolation and worthlessness! Moving on in this "health care" center, we meet Milton, tagged the resident "dirty old man." But guess what? There's no such thing as a dirty *old* man; no more so than a dirty *young* man! People like Milton, desperate for human contact, may reach out inappropriately by pinching and grabbing. Why?

When we stopped Milton's world and put him in a nursing home, he got off. For one thing, he's not ill — just minor impairments. He's in this home because his town lacks adequate home-health and other supportive services. Now committed, often oversedated, he's floundering. A misfit. As Mrs. Eleanor Blakeslee, Family Relations Counselor, has described such persons:

> "When previous standards of ethics, morality and personal cleanliness are relaxed, he resorts to excessive interest in the body and sex in an effort to recapture earlier experiences. The threat of impotence is great and may bring on psychotic episodes. Both men and women may resort to exhibitionism. The man may act out sexually to prove himself. Because he feels alone and isolated, he magnifies sexual interest."

Alone and isolated? That's it! Climb back aboard, Milton. We'll give you feedback from the world. Grabbing, you see, is simply behavior out of contact. The farther you stray from reality, having little to do or think about, the more your sex impulses get out of hand, the less you realize what is and what is not acceptable. Adult that you are, we'll give you things to do, to think about, responsibilities to help you regain confidence in yourself. Too, we will respect your wishes and rights to privacy. Soon you will have surplus respect to pass on to others. Now, will the new, will the real Mr. Milton Jones please stand up?

### Sexuality: Somebody Could Sue?

Just what is sexuality? We might call it the sum total of our being. It is that "something" which validates the wholeness of the individual. It is the acceptance of ourselves in the knowledge that "I am fearfully and wonderfully made." Sexuality is that within us which consolidates our wholeness, integrity and innate worth.

How do we uphold the sexuality of older persons? Sometimes when overeager to control, we might consider where human relating begins. Gerontologist Lester Kirchendall, Ph.D. gives us seven conditions: confidentiality, trust, empathy, mutuality of motivation, affectional (sic.) expression, emotional investment and sexual expression. When an older couple shares these values (and this does not endorse promiscuity), what if it does include the sexual embrace? Says Dr. Alexander Comfort:

> "The time may come when we are confronted with a new right. Patients don't forfeit their civil rights by having reached a certain chronological age. Nursing homes, rehabilitation centers and even hospitals will have to change their attitude about sex among patients. I think it would be possible to sue a nursing home for compromising patients' rights and I hope somebody does it!"

The bridge to human relationships is communication. It is only through the senses that we can cross this bridge. With a hearing and sight loss, half the world escapes us. Then, with diminished taste and smell, more ground is lost. Madly frustrating is the loss of speech, the inability to express oneself.

Still, there is one consolation, touch. There's always touch, the one sense which, for most people, remains intact throughout a lifetime. Small wonder, then, that many older people grab and grope for touch. Just for nearness. Just to know someone cares. As we begin to understand sensory loss, perhaps fewer persons like Jake will be led to the slaughter. It happened at 2:00 a.m.

### The Destruction of "Jake"

Making her rounds, the night nurse flashed the light on Jake's bed. It was empty. Frantically she searched. Then, from the far corridor came the cry: "He's here. Here's Jake, in bed with Bonnie!" Both were sound asleep. With a poke and a tongue-lashing, Jake was hustled back to his room, tied with restraints. "We can't have him bedhopping," cried the nurse, "what will people think!" Would you call that a *creative* solution?

This episode in the life of Mr. Jake McGuire launched him on his precipitous downhill plunge. It was on this night when, cornered, humiliated, he was sacrificed on the altar of public opinion. The next day he refused his meals. As the weeks passed, he lost interest in activities, in food, in people, in life itself. Deterioration rapidly set in. Within a month, Jake lay in his grave.

Still, we never learn. We struggle with Victorian fallout, that tragic denial of sexuality as it pertains to the long-lived. Not surprisingly, those least able to cope with our Jakes, Minnies and Miltons are their ever-loving relatives.

Marriage exists for the fulfillment of each partner as an entity and for the couple as a team. The young have no monopoly. Yet what killjoys our older lovers encounter! Relatives, now in the driver's seat, are vociferous in their objections to late-life marriage.

"I just can't imagine Grandma . . .!" or, "There are too many legal tangles."

It is true that late marriage involves economic considerations, inheritance and such. But are these tangles insurmountable? With professional counsel, with loving concern, could they be unravelled? Why *can't* we imagine Grandma, if she wants it, radiant in a new love relationship? (A pity her chances are slim. Older women outnumber the men at least three to one — a figure which rises the older they become.)

### That Sexless Sanctuary

Despite guaranteed patients' rights, why are hospitals and health-care facilities sexless sanctuaries, most of them frowning on any form of sexual expression? Why? Especially in view of well-known research by Ellis and Arbarbanel, which shows that "sex desire, even in its impaired state, is quite beneficial to the aging process. As long as it functions, interest in life persists."

### No Partner? What Then?

Constantly cropping up in congregate living, that "no partner" issue is a sticky one. It baffles the client, staff and family. In the literature, rarely is it adequately addressed, let alone discussed in staff inservice classes.** And so, to the consternation of all, situations arise which are awkwardly — no, badly handled. Right now we will pull this from under the rug for, if the patient comes first, we have to consider how best to deal with it. I refer to the common practice (among clients in congregate living settings or in their own homes) of self-stimulation, properly termed "masturbation." Here is a typical situation, involving either a man or a woman:

---

** Recommended: *Sexuality and Aging* booklet for staff and families. Published by the Andrus Gerontology Center, University of Southern California, Los Angeles, CA 90007. We also suggest that patients' relatives be invited to share in these inservie sessions. This results in greater understanding and cooperation.

For years a widower, Mr. "K" has never shown interest in seeking a new partner. "Nobody could replace my Elsie," he tells us. However, quite naturally, but to his dismay and feelings of guilt, he sometimes experiences sexual stirrings. But because his church or Victorian upbringing have ingrained in him the notion that this is wicked, he suppresses his urges.

On one particular day, however, these feelings become intense. Sitting in his wheelchair in the hall and unaware that others are around, he begins to fondle his genitals. At that moment who should wander by but Gert, of all people! Emitting a hoot, she grabs his wheelchair, roughly spins it around, "shoots" him back to his cubicle all the while scolding, shaming, mortifying him. (Time and again one sees this kind of "horrors — naughty-naughty,-look-what-he's-doing" approach!)

Now we'll look at another reaction. This time, instead of Gert, it is Annie who happened by. Mature and sensitive, she turns his chair around, gently glides it back to his room. With a non-judgmental expression on her face she says: "Mr. 'K' I'll pick you up for dinner in an hour." Softly she closes the door.

Like most of us, Annie doesn't know the perfect solution to many such situations. She does know, however, come what may, that there are two magic words she must always keep in mind. Dignity. Self-esteem. At all costs, in any situation, she must maintain the dignity and self-esteem of all patients committed to her care. And she's doing a beautiful job.

Recently I read a statistic — and don't ask me how they go about finding such information! It said that probably 98% of the world's population has at some time engaged in self-stimulation. Those of you who rear children know that it starts very early; that it has been noted even among very young babies. Again, if the patient comes first, it behooves the staff and family of patients to refrain from judgmental, destructive reactions to this kind of behavior, to seek creative solutions.

Today we have discarded the outmoded myths which taught children that "God will cut off your hand if you touch yourself," or "your hair will fall out; scars will appear on your face to give away your secret!" Such scare tactics caused pathetic feelings of guilt and worthlessness. Nobody needs that. In our society it is difficult enough to be lonely, divorced, widowed, separated. People need

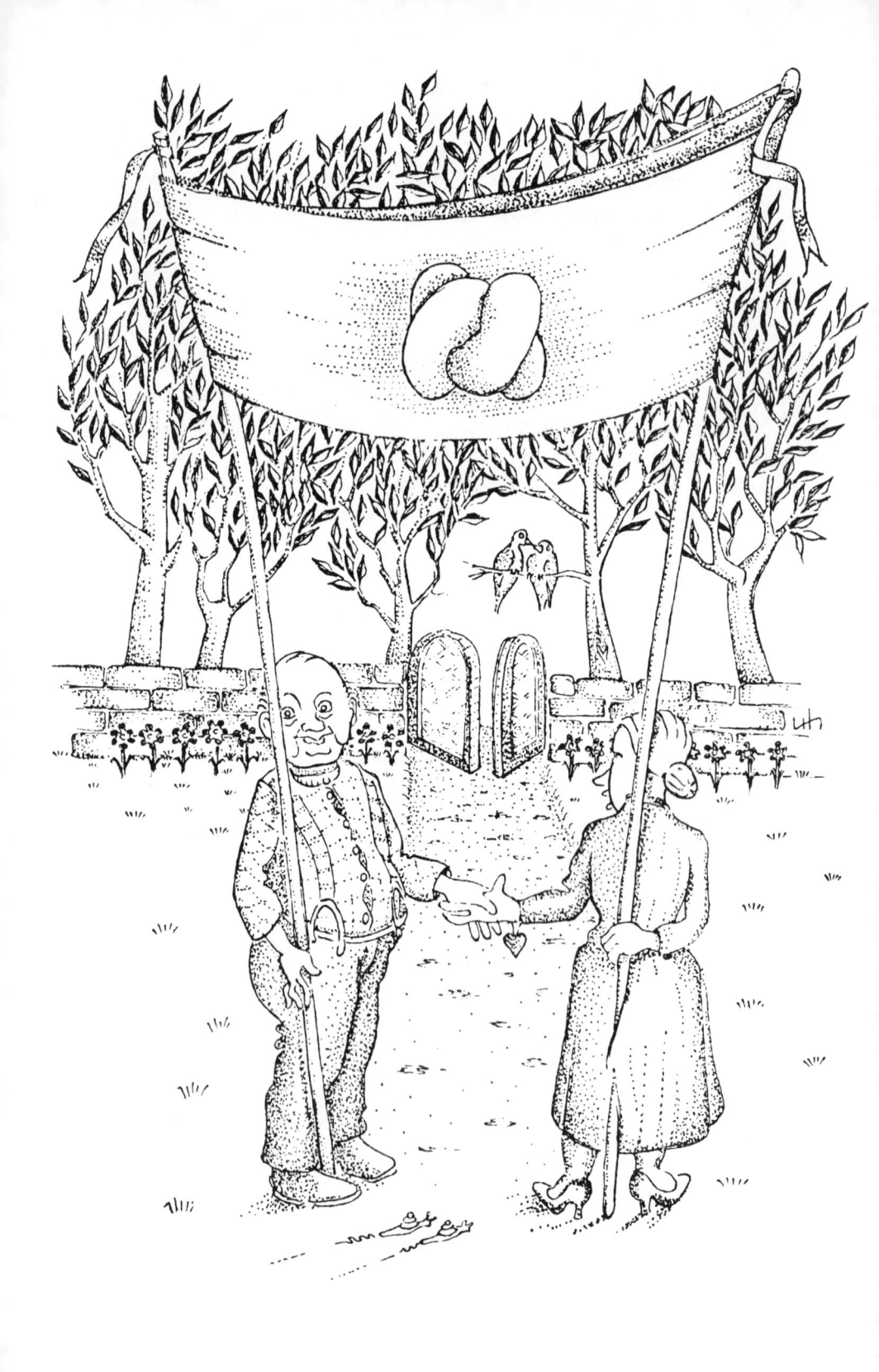

love, understanding and support. They need the "Annie" approach!

To you, the hospital or nursing home administrator, we ask: "What is the hang-up?" Fear of losing your license? Community uproar? Is it that old "what-will-people-think" routine?

People? Who's that? Just who is this mythical monster who cracks the whip over the very souls of your clients? Go slay that dragon. Make decisions less related to staff convenience and more closely applicable to the well-being of your clients.

Finally, to you good people of the Grand Generation, we uphold you as individuals of dignity and worth. We wish you love. You are free. Make your own choices — the kinds which, while respecting the rights of others, allow you privacy — a bubble of breathing space around your own person. For, after all, as you keep trying to tell us (and if we would only listen), "THE SUNSET CAN BE JUST AS BEAUTIFUL AS THE SUNRISE!"

# PART THREE: *RETIREMENT*
## Blueprint to Oblivion — or What?

*To forget one's ancestors is to be
a brook without a source, a tree without a root.*
*Chinese Proverb*

**CHAPTER TEN**

**MOTHERS'/FATHERS' DAY — IN *CHINA*?**
***Unheard of!***

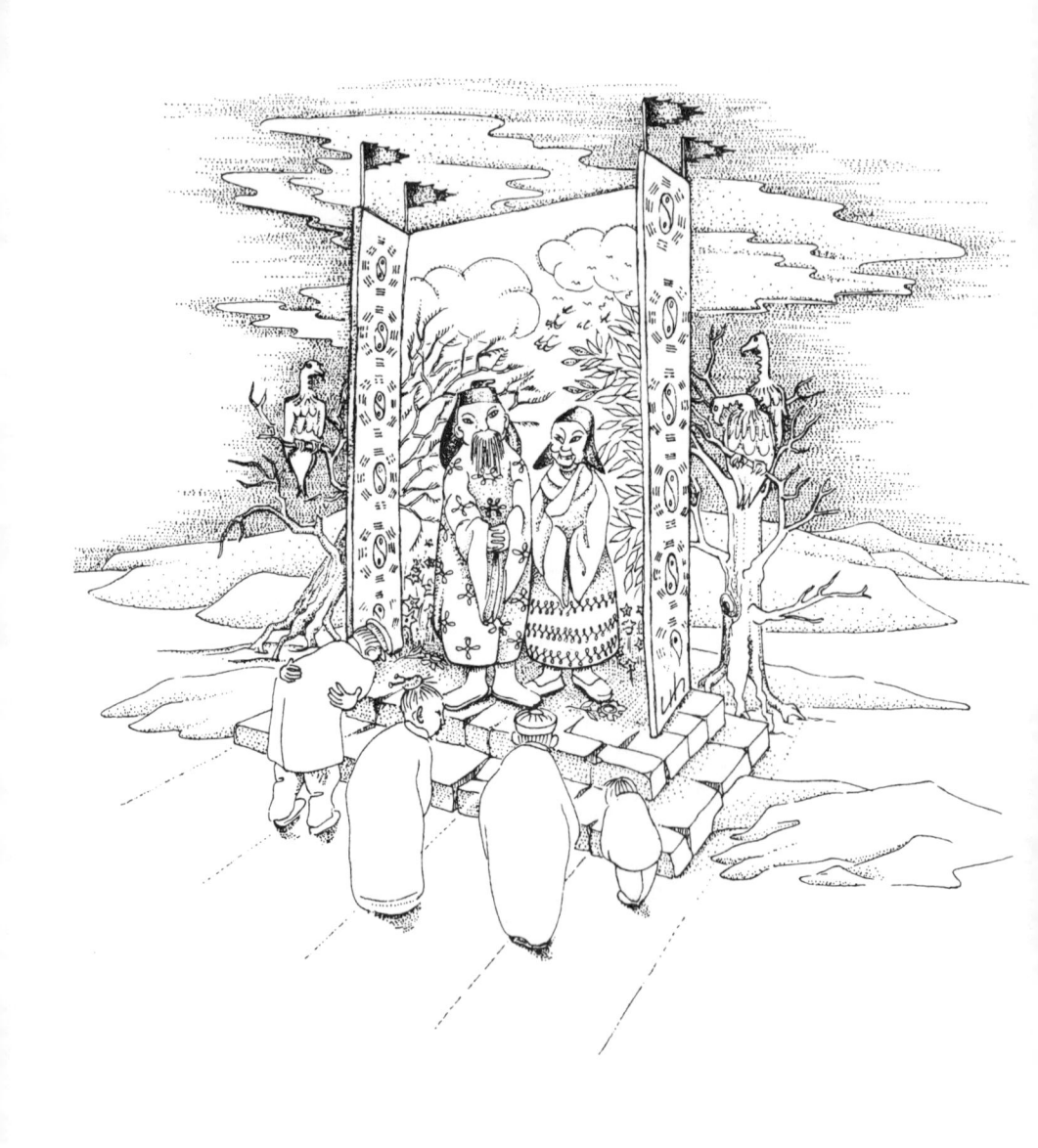

## Mothers'/Fathers' Day — in *China?* Unheard of!

*As legend has it, a woman walks down a rural path, meets an ancient farmer guiding his water buffalo and asks: "And what is your glorious age?"*
*"I am 90," he replies.*
*"Cheer up," she consoles, "the years pass swiftly. Soon you will be 95, a more honorable age. In 10 years you will be 100, a* most *honorable, venerable age!"*

After an absence of 50 years, I recently visited five major cities and some rural areas in China. Our gerontology study group, sponsored by the National Council on Aging, took a brief look at hospitals, old age homes and retirement communes. We met with Chinese gerontologists and geriatricians. After this enlightening adventure, I bring back to my country an unmistakable message concerning late life.

It was a joy to note that the old tradition, reverence for age, lives on. Greatgrandfather is King-of-the-Castle where it is not uncommon for three, sometimes even four generations to share the same home. This is changing, however, as modernization takes hold. Yet the patriarch still believes: "I have crossed more bridges than you have crossed streets so how can you young ones know the terrain?"

Since time immemorial the Chinese have worshipped their ancestors — their way of commemorating the spirits of the dead, spirits which continue to live within the family. Although in modern China, this practice is discouraged, the tradition persists. As a child growing up in central China (1917-1930), I recall my father's warning not to use a certain phrase which I had overheard during a heated quarrel between two laborers (coolies). "That phrase infuriates those who revere their forebears," he told me. It translates to: "Curses on your stinking ancestors!"

### Filial Duty — or is it Privilege?

Mothers'/Fathers' Day — in China? *Every day* is Parents' Day. Powerful — the sense of filial responsibility! And so, in that land, the modern "je-je" (grandfather) and the "nai-nai" (grandmother) feel secure within the family circle. They enjoy their "Five Guarantees," that is, rights to food, clothing, shelter, medical care and burial. (China is the world's only country which in her Constitution spells out these rights.)

Overseeing the "Five Guarantees" is the eldest, or "prime" son. If neither he nor a daughter is alive, the assignment falls on the usually willing shoulders of a grandchild. Neglect of parents can result in a prison sentence or worse. Mr. Ly, one of our guides, told us of an extreme case when, in 1981, all five sons failed to provide for their parents. The couple committed suicide. Incurring the wrath of the community, the prime son was hauled into court, sentenced to death. The execution was carried out.

Chinese posters portray this theme of reverence for age. The late-life years are regarded as a Heaven-sent blessing. By contrast, reflect a moment on the limits that we in the U.S. place on the concept of longevity. "Yes," we say, "I'd like to live a long life if . . . if . . .

> . . . if I remain mentally alert;
> . . . if I don't become "senile;"
> . . . if I don't lie there like a vegetable;
> . . . if I don't go to a nursing home."

What does this say about our culture where few Americans realize, as gerontologists point out, the vast potential for our later years? Research abounds with exciting findings — the prevention of illness, the importance of positive attitudes and continued activity, the need to explode our many misconceptions of aging. One example of today's notable research: *Memory loss is not a natural function of age!* We need to believe, as do the Chinese, that people can and should remain alert over a lifetime."*

China has its share of Alzheimer's disease and other conditions resulting in brain deterioration. But here we focus on a fact that intrigued me as we observed health care facilities — the apparent absence of "man-made senility." The Chinese believe that the golden age lies ahead, rather than behind in youth and innocence. "Yes," they say, "you *can* teach an old dog new tricks!" Rather than stepping aside, the old ones, in general, stay within the mainstream of family and community life.

### In China You Don't Retire — You Refire!

Said one retiree: "I never expected so much happiness in retirement!" In this vast land, 80 million persons over 60 could change the environment. And so they do. Although retirement is mandatory — the men at 60, the women at 50 or 55 — these people don't seem to retire at all. They refire their energies and skills. Needed by society, they perform multiple community-service functions. What do they do? I found this information in a Chinese newsletter:

A grandmother provides after-school counselling;

A retired doctor gives free medical aid in his neighborhood;

On government matters, the wisdom of the elders is sought;

A former law-enforcer assists the "Peoples' Traffic Police;"

Millions of grandparents care for the grandchildren while parents go to work;

Former welders, tea-pickers, silk-makers, jade-carvers pass on their skills to others learning the profession;

Former educators oversee remedial instruction, train new teachers; teach the unemployed;

Ten percent of retired business people devote time to improving production and management.

---

*Barring certain as yet incurable brain damage which, according to experts, afflicts no more than about six percent of our over-65 population. Much mental confusion is preventable and reversible, as noted in previous chapters.

Said one manager: "Our company was founded by people now retired. We must pay special attention to their well being, now that they are elderly."

There is little waste of people-power. On the farms, in the streets, we saw men and women of advanced age pulling heavy wagons loaded with produce. By continued activity, retirees remain functional, contributing to the nation's progress. In the past 35 years, that progress has been phenomenal. For example, life expectancy has soared. In 1949 it was age 35. Today it nears 70. China's improved methods of sanitation, their standard of living has made giant strides. Old and young — all contribute to the nation's goals.

Although their standard of living nowhere approaches that of the U.S., their advances have been astounding. One cannot compare modern China with modern America. Understanding comes by comparing the old with the new China. As a child living over there, then returning 50 years later, I can do some comparing. The changes I saw were nothing short of amazing.

In the 1920s, people were dropping dead by the millions, literally, from famine, floods, and disease. Beggars displayed their self-inflicted wounds to entice passers-by to toss them a penny. I remember riding a rickshaw pulled by a coolie and coming upon a beggar who had stretched himself full length across the narrow street. Without hesitating the coolie pulled my rickshaw clear over the prostrate body, never looking back. Nobody seemed surprised.

In the 1920s my father was chairman of the China Famine Relief Committee. In appreciation, Dr. Sun Yat Sen, China's first president, presented him with a medal depicting the "Order of the Felicitous Grain." Today this medal hangs on my living room wall.

And oh, back then, the swarms of flies! So many, in fact, that our Chinese cook "Da Tze Fu" often handed me a fly-swatter, saying: "Lanshi (Nancy) I'll give you a penny for every 100 flies you swat in the kitchen!" What youngster wouldn't fall for that!

Rarely, today, does one see a fly or a beggar. Not all, but most citizens have enough to eat. It is claimed that no person under age 40 is illiterate today. However, serious overpopulation problems still exist, dispite the birth-contrtol clinics despite the one-child-to-a-family pledge couples must sign. Due to peasant protests, China is slowly backing off from her rigid population control policy in rural areas. Another problem, infanticide, makes a difference in population count.**

Age in action? We saw that old people themselves are the very ones who inspect old age homes. Logical! Who better to evaluate what the long-lived person wants!

### The House of Respect

Old age homes, known as the "House of Respect" or "Homes for Respected Elderly" do exist, yet the very concept of such institutions is alien to their culture. They ask: "How can personal services and devotion of adoring children be replaced by paid personnel?"*** However, as China has become increasingly industrialized, the old age home has become a necessity. To be eligible for admission, a person must:

1) Have no close relatives

2) Be financially dependent (although some pay out of their pensions.)

3) Be willingly admitted. (If not willing, the elder is cared for by neighbors assigned to help with meals, cleaning, etc.)

As for comfort, sanitation and decor, China can learn from the U.S. We visited facilites which were just plain cold, the indoor temperature hovering around 55 degrees Fahrenheit. Not even the 101-year-old man who hugged some of us seemed to mind the chill. Indoors as well as outdoors, residents wear the traditional multi-layered padded clothing, warm caps and mittens. I suspect that having been hardened all their lives, they catch fewer colds than do we Westerners in our overheated dwellings.

Bathrooms in old age homes are few and far between and, by our standards, primitive. There was only one TV for an entire floor. Cubicles contained pot-bellied stoves. I saw no activities rooms, such as we know them. They have other ideas. Residents keep active by sweeping their own rooms, setting tables, making

---

**Chinese data indicate that infanticide is high, a loss of about 60,000 baby girls a year. (From the International Herald Tribune, July 12, 1984.)

***The situation differs in the U.S. in that we are a more mobile society in which parents and adult children often live miles apart. We also have more employment of women.

beds, doing laundry, caring for dogs, cats, goats and pigs — jobs which in the U.S. would violate our sacrosanct rules and regulations. For a Chinese ambulatory resident to sit around, do nothing and be waited on — unthinkable! No time to stare at walls, complain, develop imaginary ailments, hit you with a cane for attention, swallow sedatives indiscriminately, suffer insomnia. What a colossal lesson for many U.S. nursing homes!

Those were the "intermediate care" patients. What about the bedridden? We saw just one ward of 16 beds. Of this group, only one patient appeared to me to be "out of it." Brief observation revealed that all the rest were sharp, shiney-eyed people who shook our hands vigorously.

"How do you do it?" I asked an attending nurse. "How do these bedfast persons, despite severe disabilities, remain so alert?"

Her answer, in fairly good English, surprised me not at all for by now I had drawn my own conclusions. "Ah," she replied, "action is the key. This home is not isolated. School kids drop in constantly to learn wisdom from these elders. Relatives, friends, volunteers keep up a constant stream of visitations, bringing in musical instruments, games, puppet-shows, babies, animals, magazines." And then she added: "A local baker donates goodies; a restaurant chef provides gifts of specialties; grain stores donate rice. So you see, here there is always a 'buzz' of activity to keep them alert and interested in life. It's like in New York City — your Grand Central Station!"

Some other fascinating observations: Aides and orderlies are carefully screened *according to their devotion to the aged.* They receive six months training before they may begin work. Residents receive the finest food available, with choices from a host of delicacies piled in bowls all over the table. Doctors visit twice a week here, although in one rural old age home we visited there was a doctor in residence. I asked one doctor: "What would happen if you were to neglect or withhold treatment from a patient?" His quick response: "I would incur the wrath of the patient, his friends and from every staff member in this place!"

Obviously, all these activities described were not part of a devised "Care Plan." Not ordered by a doctor for "therapeutic" reasons. The whole approach was a natural spin-off of their regular life style. On second thought, that's no surprise. What else could one expect from a Chinese *Home for Respected Aged?*

## A Sense of Belonging

By the second week of our tour we were getting a feel for their way of life, not just from observation but from hearing gerontologists who lectured us formally and chatted with us informally. We saw that their lives, though from our standpoint materialistically meagre, seemed content, uncomplicated. Contributing to good health is the fact that everybody rides bicycles, young, middle-aged and old. (Some very old ones ride tricycles.) Nobody owns a car — only state officials. Swarms of bikes in the streets, everyone riding to work, to market, to the shops. Nobody worries about the latest car model or keeping up status. And trying to cross a street in any large city like Shanghai, having to weave in and out among bicycles, you almost sacrifice your life! And how delightful those traffic cops, perched high on covered platforms in the center of intersections! The way cyclists ignore their signals, you wonder how they keep their cool.

Considering their national goals of rapid modernization, we wonder how the Chinese feel inwardly about governmental domination. Outwardly they seem so serene. I think of this country as a giant tapestry in the making, each citizen weaving his allotted spot so as not to leave a hole. Dedication to a "great cause" certainly never hurt a person's mental health!

Of course, as visiting professionals, we were aware that our short stay (packed as it was with new experiences, data and gerontological insights) did not make us experts on the overall China aging scene. We saw only a small part, one selected for us by authorities. But I came away more certain than ever that *one of the most dangerous treatments for the long-lived is enforced inactivity.* The Chinese have much to teach us.

On our homebound flight from Hong Kong I wondered: "Can we learn something from them about acceptance of age? Are we ever, without resorting to denials and cosmetic coverups, to grasp the idea of aging with grace, viewing late life as an honorable estate, even admitting we are headed towards a 'glorious age?'

Now that I've been back to China, absorbing the "aura" of their culture, this does something to me. Makes me want to philosophize!

Life is an upward journey. We climb, coming ever closer to the top of a mountain where at last we attain that coveted, honorable status, old age. As we go, we gather up learning and wisdom. We try to keep our hearts unwrinkled, our minds alert, our spirits alive to the fragrance and fullness of the world about us. Finally, reaching the summit, drinking in the panorama of life stretched before us, we feel oneness with nature, with the Universe, with our Creator.

Walking in the footsteps of those who have gone before, we now understand, at last, what they in their late life have endured. We see them now in a softer light. No longer do we think of them as unproductive. Oh no. They produce all right. Not things like money or commodities. They produce love, wisdom, empathy, joy, understanding.

What a heritage! It's now in our grasp. We will pass it all on to those who, still climbing, follow in our path.

Oh, America, we need more than just that *annual* Mothers'/Fathers' day! Make that, Chinese style, an *everyday* celebration.

Growing old, aging serenely?

Confucius say: "Watch the experts — one fortnight in China worth thousand gerontology textbooks!"

*A Troublesome Trend in
U.S. Advertising*

**CHAPTER ELEVEN**

**THOSE MAGAZINE ADS**
**Take a Hard Look**

## Those Magazine Ads Take a Hard Look*

Flip the pages of your latest gerontology/geriatrics magazine. Here's a full-page ad featuring an aging patient. The caption reads: "Disturbed and Disruptive." Here's another one. An unshaven, mean-looking old man bears the label: "Assaultive." Now turn to an earlier issue and note that older woman — oh so nervous and agitated! Or that fist-pounding "monster," who, as the ad stresses in big red letters, is guilty of "tantrums." Here's a slouched, depressed old woman who is saying: "I'm too much trouble to keep at home." (Yes, she *is* unless the daughter wises up and zonks her with the drug being promoted!) And here's a photo of grandfather who, having upset the family at the dinner table, marches out the door, good and mad!

A troublesome trend in U.S. advertising. But it goes even further. Some companies are so bold as to transform the adjective "geriatric" into a noun. Presto! It's magic! Suddenly all elders become *"geriatrics!"* (What *would* Mr. Webster say?) Well, I

*Originally published in "Geriatric Care" Eymann Publications, Box 3577, Reno, NV 89505.

know what *I* would say. "Listen you," I'd holler, "when I'm old, don't call me a "geriatric" or I'll call you an "obstetric" or a "pediatric" or a "cardiac!" That way we'll *all* become nobodies.

Now how about this patronizing ad — an angelic, "cute" little old lady murmuring: "I made a flower today!" (Substitute her face for that of a first grader dutifully reporting to her parents.) And while we're noting how ads can "infantize," note this one, the ultimate in degradation. It spotlights the "diapered" buttocks of an aging woman. Now tell me. Did the model give informed consent? Or, unaware of cameras, was she sedated? We will form a picket line around the next advertiser who applies the word "diaper" to dignified adults or who otherwise demeans that generation.

By contrast, turn to any youth-glorifying magazine. Find a cigarette ad. Here's one — a photo of a majestic mountain with the caption: "COME TO MARLBORO COUNTRY." Any negativism? No way. You won't find a horseback rider depicted as skinny, jaundiced, baggy-panted or, slouching in the saddle, dead drunk!

Now flip over to a perfume-promoting ad. Will you find that model portrayed as obese, agitated, assaultive or disruptive? Youth we worship. But age? Despite the wisdom, the maturity, we tolerate negative portrayals.

Subtly or overtly, deliberately or thoughtlessly, our media wields the power to trample on the sensibilities of mature people. True, we *do* have elders who are agitated, disturbed or unshaven. But such charcteristics are equally represented in those of every other age group.

At a time when health professionals are accentuating the positives of longevity, these ads tear them down. More seriously, they wreak havoc on the self esteem of elders. How do *your* grandparents react to an ad which degrades their whole generation?

You caregivers, you families of aging persons, don't allow those ads to go unchallenged. Think what they say to foreigners about U.S. societal attitudes! (Imagine one of those ads appearing in a Chinese or Portuguese publication!)

Of course, you will find other types of ads — those which are supportive. Here, for example, I see one that is respectful of the "Grand Generation." It shows a well-groomed, shiny-eyed old woman and bears the caption: "Helping the nursing home patient

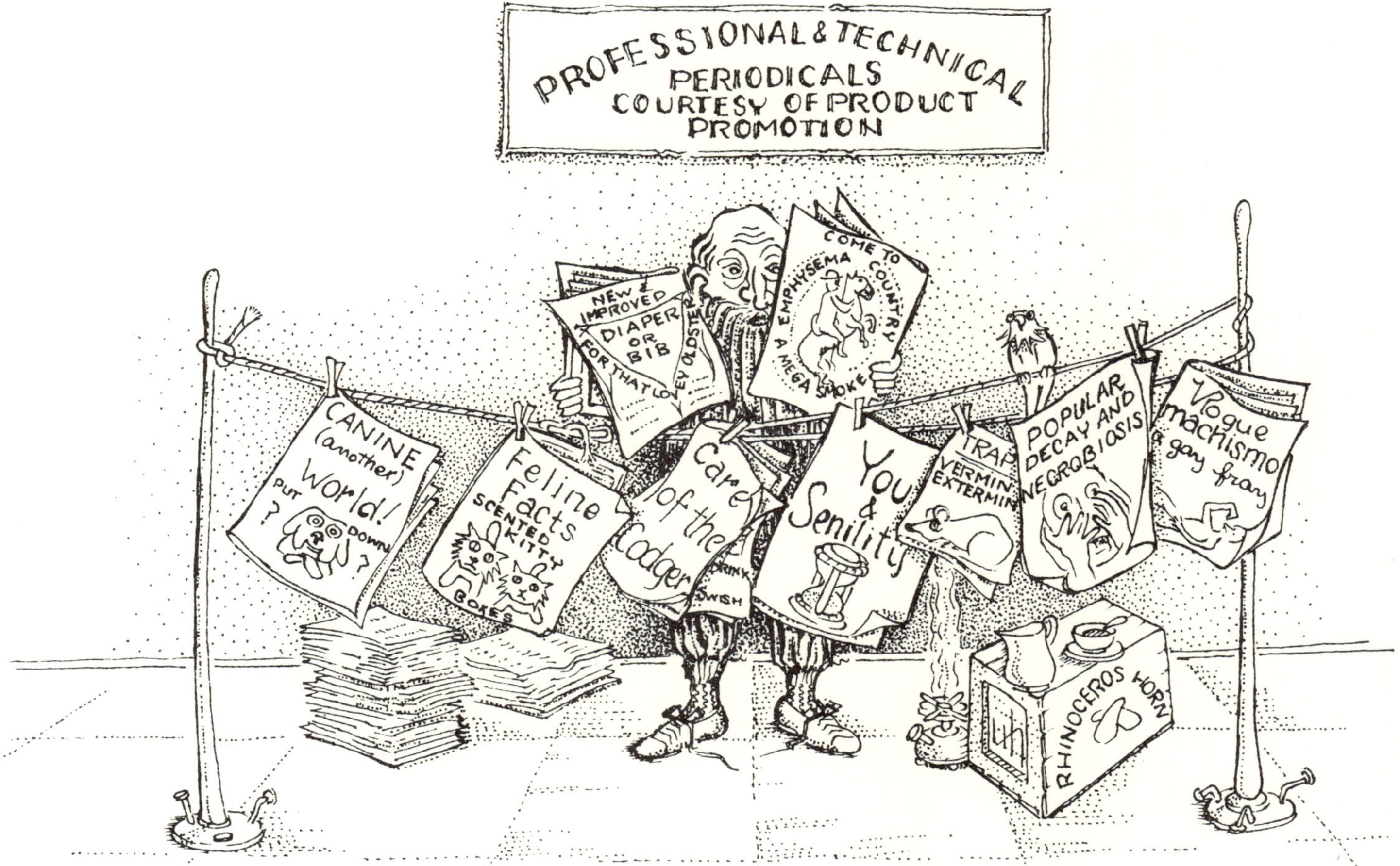
PROFESSIONAL & TECHNICAL PERIODICALS COURTESY OF PRODUCT PROMOTION
NEW & IMPROVED DIAPER OR BIB FOR THAT LOVEY OLDSTER
COME TO EMPHYSEMA COUNTRY A MEGA SMOKE
CANINE (another) World! PUT DOWN ? ?
Feline Facts SCENTED KITTY BOXES
Care of the Codger
DRINK SWISH
You & Senility
TRAP VERMIN EXTERMIN
POPULAR DECAY AND NECROBIOSIS
Vogue machismo a gay fray
RHINOCEROS HORN

to be active and involved."

But for those others, my friends, what can be done?

March on those magazines. Swamp them with protest cards. Hit them where it hurts — in the pocketbook. Tell them that unless they update their ads and the attitudes that prompted them, you will not only cancel your subscription, you'll boycott their product. Advertisers must champion the dignity of those who "have come a little further in the experience of life."

Today, our nation strives towards greater humanization of our health care institutions. As increasingly we become sensitized to the rights of the long-lived, get out there and remind the advertiser who he is, what his function is. Does he not represent a liason between his product and the trends of the nation? In that case, he had jolly well better know *both* before he can effectively serve either!

*Like June, why isn't **Home Health Care**
"bustin' out all over?"*


## CHAPTER TWELVE


## DON'T RUSH THE ROCKING CHAIR!

## Don't Rush the Rocking Chair!

I am growing older. As you are. All of us aging gracefully, of course, like that 74-year old who, hearing a wolf-call, quipped:

>That whistle when I hear it now
>Serves only to remind me
>That probably a pretty girl
>Is walking right behind me!

We've lived to the hilt, haven't we! But now retired, it's time for our return match with life. Granted we have an ache or two, slight or severe, but perk up! There appears to be no mental decline with age.

Hard to believe? Ask Dr. James Birren of the Andrus Gerontology Center, UCLA. "Responses come slower," he says, "but in healthy persons . . . high mental competence through the octo- and nonogenarian years." He should know. He's studied the aging brain for 40 years.

If that's not enough, ask Dr. Robert Butler, renown aging expert who says: "In general, with good physical and mental health, adequate educational levels and intellectual stimulation, it appears there is not the decline in intellectual abilities with age, as was previously thought. In fact, some abilities increase, such as judgment, accuracy and general knowledge."

High mental competence through the 80s? Like my friend Mrs. Evelyn Hobday who at age 83 takes flying lessons? Like Mrs. Brandon, 94, who for 43 years has taken a pre-dawn swim — in the nude? Like Mr. Harley, 85, who bakes 600 fruit cakes a year? High expectations of yourself — that helps a whole lot!

You know what our problem *really* is? Although other nations tell us that age is beautiful, we accept our society's image of ourselves — that we are "over the hill," or we've "had it," or we're "falling apart." Fiddle! We've just come a little farther in the experience of life.

So you think you'll land in a nursing home? Guess again. Surprise! Only five percent of those over 65 land in such places. (Many may spend some temporary time, however, in an institution.) So you expect to become "senile?" (ghastly word!) Relax. Again, watch your expectations. We've said it in other chapters, but remember for all time — most who become confused are suffering reversible, preventable conditions, often culturally produced from lack of environmental, intellectual stimulation. Your chances of remaining mentally alert, *if you work at it,* are excellent. You move a muscle to keep it strong. Move your *brain* every day. Do challenging things! Get with good nutrition. (Watch those French fries, chocolates, cokes and cholesterol-laden no-no's.)

Then why the nonsense that America needs more and bigger nursing homes? And how come they, instead of Home Health Services, are "bustin' out all over?" Sure the aging population is puffing up like a balloon. But whoa, America! We're riding a runaway horse. Look who's profiting. "It's the logical answer," say the nursing home and building industries, "to an expanding older population."

Or *is* it? Here's a pin. Let's puncture that premise.

How many institutionalized clients do not belong there, were inappropriately admitted in the first place, unnecessarily kept there when improved? Estimates range from 20 to 40%. Too high. Although today more care is taken to screening applicants, there are loopholes. What's Mrs. "Clark" doing in that health care facility? Nobody at home to bathe her — can't let her son do it!

Make no mistake. A good nursing home is a blessing for those who really need concentrated care. But for the others? Hold your hat! In the U.S. hundreds of thousands could remain in their own homes if communities like yours would step up the alternatives. I call them "stepping stones to the institution," supports which would prevent or postpone the giant leap direct to the institution.

Urgent! (And for this I have been pleading for 20 years!) *We need more, we need adequate, we need drastic expansion of community services.* Let's quit footdragging. Let's catch up with many European countries which are more farsighted than we. Let's check that runaway horse with:

HOME HEALTH AGENCIES IN EVERY TOWN AND HAMLET IN THE U.S.

HOMEMAKERS' SERVICES everywhere.

MEALS-ON-WHEELS, seven days a week and on holidays. Volunteer to eat with the lonely recipients of these meals.

DAY CARE SERVICES — horrendously scarce, but essential.

SENIOR BUSES, all with hydraulic lifts and ramps.

HANDYMAN SERVICES (on call for lawn mowing, storm window installing, and to do errands, etc.)

DAILY TELEPHONE CONTACT for every homebound person.

RESPITE SERVICES in every town for the caregiver.

DELIVERIES (of books, groceries, etc. in every locale).

THERAPISTS to make home calls everywhere.

PHYSICIANS, DENTISTS to make housecalls. A great revival is needed. And FOSTER HOMES, next best thing to your own home, licensed and properly managed.

Whew! Look at the employment all this would generate!

"But we *have* all these in our community," you say? Yes, you probably have some of these. But check it out. What small percentage of the local need do they cover?

Meet Mr. Marks. Today he made the giant leap from home to institution. Alas, he was not among those given an alternative choice. Why not? Why, in his town do these "stepping stones" fall short?

*First,* because people do not speak up. Except for some advocate groups, like the Gray Panthers, AARP (American Association of Retired Persons), or N.C.O.A. (National Council on the Aging), we

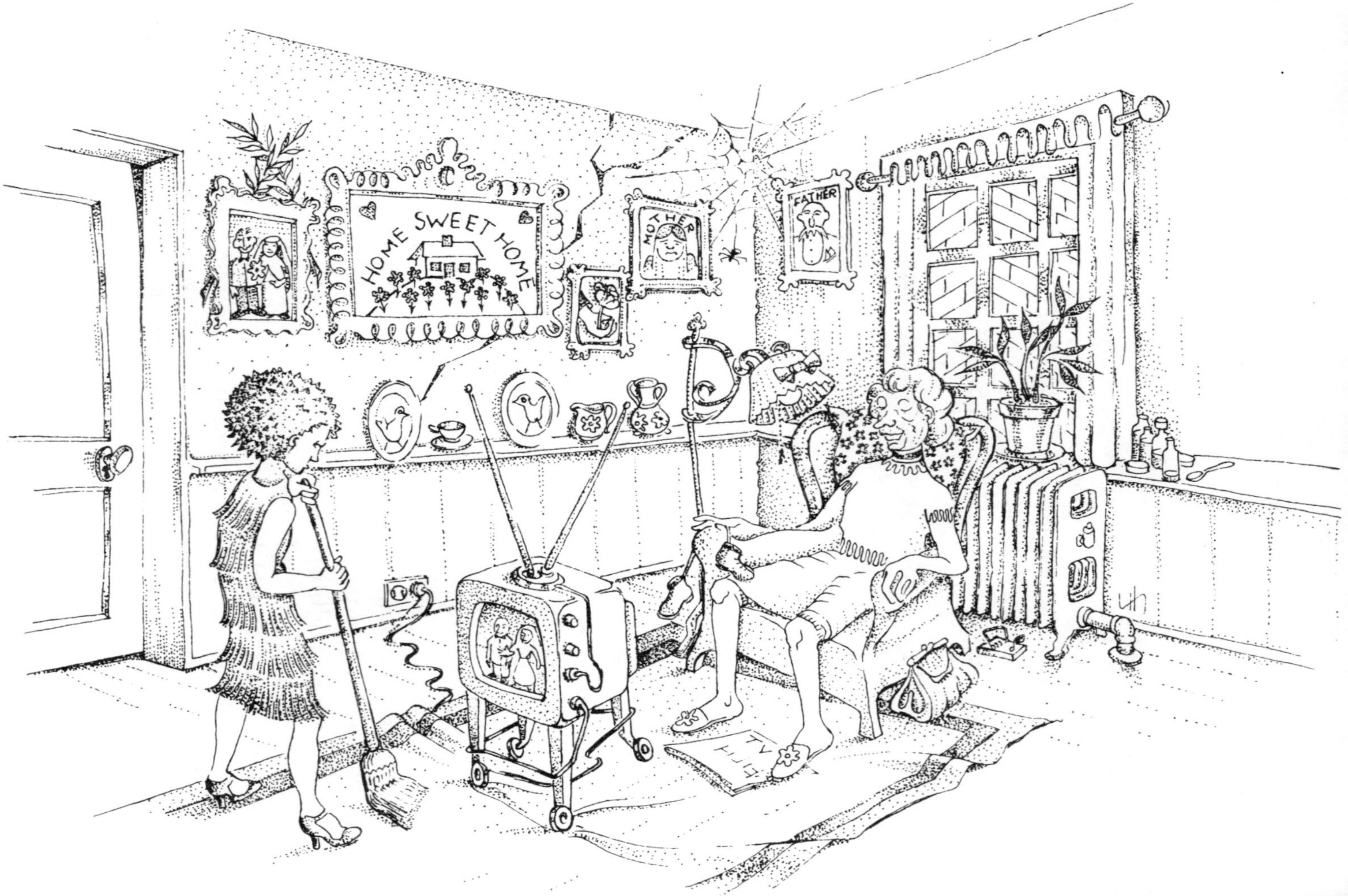
HOME SWEET HOME
MOTHER
FATHER
TV

do not voice the urgency of our need. We'd never picket City Hall or the Health Department or write to our legislators!

*Secondly*, city and government officials are dragging their feet in studying the cost savings of keeping people in their own homes.

*Compare:*

---

### HOME HEALTH CARE
Hiring nurses, aides, homemakers, etc. plus rounding up volunteers, bringing in therapists, doctors into the home
### VERSUS
### INSTITUTIONALIZATION
Building costly facilities, adding wings periodically, high staffing costs, operating overhead, rising rates for nursing home beds, environmental maintenance, utility costs, etc. . . .

---

Oh, America, how rapidly you're becoming one vast, sprawling, bursting nursing home when so many could, so many want to remain in their own homes! Filling beds rather than filling needs. So many patients in institutions receiving care beyond their actual need! Mr. Marks could have stayed in his own home, thus freeing a nursing home bed for a bona-fide invalid. But so goes the Great American Myth — that nursing homes, *unlimited,* are God's Gift to the Grand Generation!

Other nations have other notions. For them, the Care Home is the last resort. In England, Holland, Scandanavia — only two to three percent compared to our over five percent living in institutions. Their secret? Full steam ahead with alternatives in virtually every community. Huge savings in nursing home costs. Their elderly are grateful. In the U.S. how many millions of dollars a year could be saved? How can the U.S. afford NOT to go all out for these services to keep people home, where they would prefer to remain? Time for us to get this priority on the road.

*A Word of Caution:* While many home-health programs are operated efficiently and are doing a fine job, take warning from others which have met with trouble. Aides fail to show up. Backup personnel is lacking. Clients' personal belongings disappear. Help is given spasmodically, sloppily, half-heartedly. The client is left unattended, disappointed, frustrated. As in any program, strict rules must be enforced. Home Health Care and all the services it entails must be managed like any well-run business: It must be:

1) Operated by skilled personnel

2) Applicants to go into homes must be screened and bonded.

3) A dignified pay scale must be offered. (The self-respect of the worker has everything to do with performance.)

4) Continuing education for all employees must be mandatory. (Focusing on physical and psycho-social needs of the elderly or handicapped of any age.)

Don't send someone into my own private home who, with no sense of mission, is irresponsible, immature. I shouldn't have to stand for that any more than I stand for a dentist who doesn't know a molar from a bicuspid.

Beginning with the very young in our schools, teachers must instill respect for age. Gerontology* must be incorporated in school and college courses. This is the wave of the future. Our entire society — our economy, media, advertising, elections — all will be dominated by the influence of older persons who are gaining in numbers and clout. From about 13% today, in another generation they may constitute 20% of our population. "Youth cult," so long!

Meanwhile, retirees have a whale of a job to do. Keep yourself out of a nursing home. Stay alert, active, heed the words of that great humanitarian, Dr. Ethel Percy Andrus, founder of AARP**, with a membership today of 18 million persons:

*"We have a responsibility in retirement to keep ourselves well informed; to cooperate with programs that will make our nation strong morally, spiritually and materially for the benefit of all Americans."*

To that I add: We have a responsibility to keep ourselves out of that rocking chair; to preserve high mental competence through life-long learning. Look around. It's exciting to see in the modern classroom those heads of white and grey. It's the trend. Remember feisty old George Bernard Shaw? When asked: "Why, at the age of 92, are you taking up the study of Greek?" he quipped: "Why my good sir, it's now or never!"

Uppermost in your mind, isn't it — how to stay out of an institution? Personally, I prefer my own cozy bed, my own bathroom

---

*Gerontology refers to the multi-disciplinary science concerned with the aging process from the sociological, psychological, social and other approaches. It is the science of understanding pesonal and social adjustments in later life; of learning how to relate them to each other and to other aspects of life. On the other hand, *geriatrics* refers to the medical treatment of the aged. (From the Greek words "gero" - old man, and "iatrike," - medical treatment).

**American Association of Retired Persons.

with the magazine rack right *there*. I adore my cuddly cats, "Fuzzball" and "Tabbyoca," and my Husky, "China Girl." And how I love my little window to the east where "the sun come peeping in at morn!" Most of all, I cherish my independence. To keep me that way, just give me my shot, zip me up, clean my house and, with meals-on-wheels, I'll manage just fine, thank you.

*Please,* please, don't ship me needlessly, inappropriately, prematurely to a "health care center." Don't rush that rocking chair. And just because I sat on my glasses, don't presume "senility." (Remember when 16-year-old Johnny lost the car keys, you didn't label *him* senile!) We all do dumb things all our lives!

Someone said: "Love is that approach which brings to a person and to his situation the greatest benefit of good." For us older Americans; for those of us who may, at any age, be challenged by a handicap, the "greatest benefit" will come through comprehensive "Keep-us-Home" services covering all bases in the land. And then, from our Home-Sweet-Home and with grateful arms around you, we shall smile and say:

> Age is the top of a mountain high
> Clearer the air, and blue
> A long hard climb
> A bit of fatigue, but oh —
> What a wonderful view!

**PART FOUR:** *A SOCIETAL ISSUE*
 . . . **of the Stickiest Kind**

*Pretend it's you!*

## CHAPTER THIRTEEN

## *EUTHAN* . . . OR *DYSTHAN-ASIA?*

## *Euthan . . .* or *Dysthan*-asia?*

Surely each of us wants a painless, peaceful and dignified death in familiar surroundings and in the presence of those we love. This ideal is described by the word "euthanasia," from the Greek *eu*, meaning good, and *thanatos*, meaning death.

But what exactly is a good death? Let me tell you about one which will occur within the next few hours.

### Friday Afternoon, 2:00 P.M.

Here in her home, death is claiming my 82-year-old Aunt Augusta. I am now holding her hand, speaking quiet words of reassurance. For three years, Augusta has been in and out of the hospital. She suffered many strokes. Now a final CVA brings on more paralysis, helplessness. I rush to make the emergency call. I stop short. Why? *Must* she again be subjected to tubes, needles, drugs, suction machines — all those scientific marvels she so dreads? In an institution our Augusta would again be distributed among staff — everybody's, yet nobody's patient. It's that impersonal system under which medical care is generally administered

---

*This chapter, in condensed form, was published in the Nancy Fox book: *How to Put Joy into Geriatric Care*. Here, by request, it is reprinted in expanded form.

to the terminally ill.

I ask her sister: "Do you want her to re-enter the hospital?"

"NO!" comes the emphatic reply. "Here Augusta knows the touch of your hand, the sound of your voice, the one-to-one nearness which has meant security." Relieved, I see the decision is made. We will keep her at home for the remainder of her time.

It is not easy to watch Augusta's temperature spike to 104 degrees; to see the precipitous drop in her blood pressure. Moistening her lips and repositioning her, I stand by as she slides into an exhausted sleep. I recall the time she said so earnestly: "Nancy, in case of a crisis, let me remain at home."

### 4:00 P.M.

Augusta is now awakening Her skin is hot, but she is calm. It is good that she has emotional support in her final human experience. I wipe her brow. She gently presses my hand, telling me what her aphasic sounds cannot convey; that she is all right, content and under no strain, even with the knowledge that she is dying. Her dignity and humanness are preserved. Fortified by a devoted sister and being at home where she feels loved, she is being spared weeks or months of unnecessary anguish which might have resulted from the artificial lengthening of her life.

### 4:45 P.M.

And now, Augusta, your breathing becomes irregular. Your heart is tired, making its last effort. It would be unkind if, at this late stage, I were to feel your pulse or flaunt before you a cold stethoscope. Instead, I am putting my arm around your shoulder, holding you tight, helping you to cross the threshold. It won't be long now.

### 5:00 P.M.

Augusta, your lips and mouth are again becoming dry. It's not too late to swab them gently one more time. Do I discern an almost imperceptible smile, as if you were trying to tell me this helps a little bit?

### 5:10 P.M.

Your minutes are numbered, Augusta. I bid you farewell, knowing that you have been helped to embark on your journey. Yours will be a calm passage. Those of us you leave behind are grateful that you are experiencing a "good death." Your years of anguish will soon be replaced by release and repose. As I watch you lie there, your soft white hair draped over the pillow, I see that you are at peace, for you know you are not alone. You have your God. I will keep my vigil until the very end.

### 5:11 P.M.

And now, Augusta, I see the last vestige of color draining from your cheeks. You have only a minute or so more. Yet I continue to reflect — this is a good, this is a perfect death. This is euthanasia in the true, in the responsible sense of the word.

### 5:12 P.M.

Your time is now, Augusta. This is it. A deep breath. A heavy sigh. You take your final breath. Your heart stops. It is over.

Rest in peace, our beloved Augusta. Your light perpetual will shine, will always shine, here in your home.

### What is Passive Euthanasia?

The aim of passive euthanasia is to allow death to come gently. Supportive measures are not used to prolong the dying process where there is irreversible brain damage and intractable pain. Medications are given to eliminate pain, even if they tend to shorten the dying process. Passive euthanasia means *letting the person go,* rejecting anything that adds to discomfort.

### What About the Quality of Life?

One definition of death states that when cerebral function has ceased the person is dead, no matter how much spontaneous and vital function remains. Too often we overemphasize the importance of mere existence. Our society has condoned "dysthanasia," (Greek for bad, ill, difficult death) believing that everything must be done to extend a life, regardless of the cost in suffering, grief, emotional strain and financial cost. Is it really humane to maintain our terminally ill, forcing them to live in a lonely, vegetative state? Although nearly 80% of terminal patients die in hospitals, the public today is becoming increasingly aware that there exist alternatives to the "cold care" provided in countless hospital settings. Today there is HOSPICE. This mission of mercy stresses the psychological needs of both patient and family. It attaches great importance to pain control; it provides meaningful programs either in the hospice or home setting. Here is an alternative which allows for striking improvements, for appropriate, responsible care of the terminally ill.

### Euthanasia? Are There Religious Objections?

For Protestants and Roman Catholics and others, the great Easter message is that "the end of man is not the death of the body but the vision of God." Pope Pius XII said that in certain circumstances it is justifiable to refrain from using "extraordinary means." Our Judeo-Christian heritage places supreme value on the wholeness of a person, which encompasses his mental, physical and spiritual oneness as a human being of dignity and worth.

When terminal illness cancels all but the shell, surely the continuation, through machines and drugs is a *gross violation of him as a person.* Nurses know that people fear the lonely, long-drawn-out process of dying more than death itself. When social and psychological death has already occurred, his desire is then, for merciful release brought about by his biological death.

### And Then, the Doctor's Dilemma

In April, 1984, Dr. Julius Hackenthal, of West Germany, provoked a national debate over medical ethics by admitting on TV he helped a 69-year-old commit suicide.* The doctor was convinced that the stage had been reached where doctors have a duty actively, but indirectly, to help people die. The woman, her face eaten by cancer, her body scarred by 13 operations, said on film that the disease had caused her so much suffering she *wanted* to die. The doctor made sure that the release she wanted was left by the bedside for her to consume.

This raises a charged question. Should not society support our doctors as humanitarians as well as skilled technicians? They should not be held legally responsible for failure to prolong every life indiscriminately. We must speak up for legislation allowing a decison-making group (such as doctor, lawyer, clergyperson if desired, and immediate family), to relieve the individual of total responsibility.

### Opening the Doors

Thanatology deals with the social and emotional problems of dying. For too long this subject has been taboo in family discussions. Adult children of aging parents often refuse to participate, or

---

*International Herald Tribune, April 1984.

THE CHALLENGE WARD

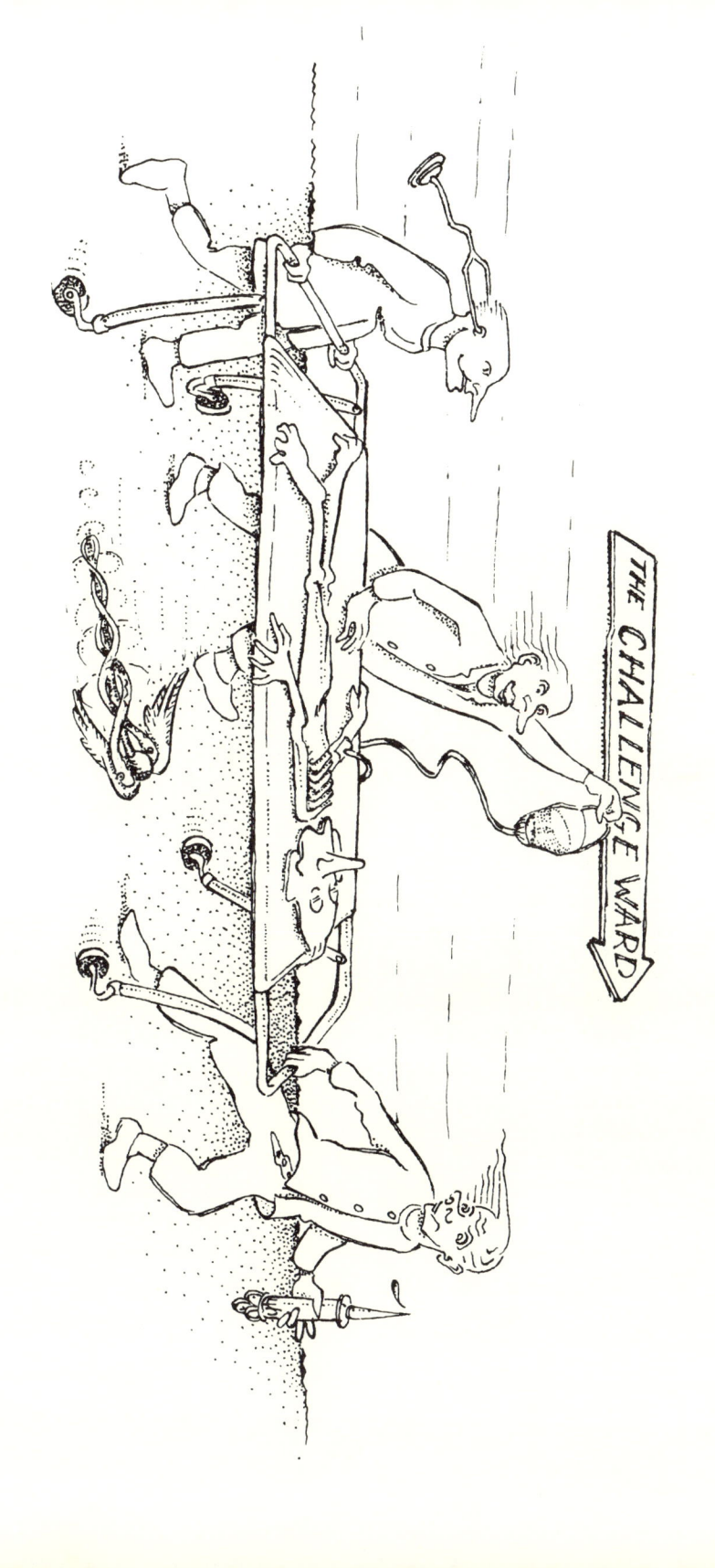

their response is superficial when asked to consider and plan the parent's death and funeral. "Oh, Ma, you'll outlive the whole bunch of us!" Closing the subject forever, an emotional gap is created.

Colleges, high schools, medical and nursing schools must make room in their curricula for thanatology. We need to read, talk about death as a natural part of the life cycle. We talk about natural birth, puberty, menopause, old-age crises, but dying and death? Understanding the final stages of life can help us, help our children deal with our innermost feelings. We must remove the mantle of mystery, apprehension, the taboos that surround the subject. With the aid of agencies such as Hospice, Home Health or Mental Health, people find that they can gain support and accept the responsibility of allowing their terminally ill relative to die serenely at home. A good birth, a good life, and now, for Augusta, a good death. Her cycle has reached completion.

### What Would I Want?

Looking ahead, I plan to maintain my positive outlook. However, practicing the art of "visualization," I can project myself as an old lady, possibly in chronic agony, stripped of dignity, faced with an intolerable, terminal disease. If I can I will speak up for merciful release. If I can't, I have (in the bottom drawer of my desk) my LIVING WILL, signed at a time when I was competent and rational. *I expect my loved ones and my doctor to take this document seriously.* My right to integrity will not be undermined. I will not be reduced to a mechanically ventilated and circulated shell. I will expect you to let me go. LET ME GO. Are you listening? LET ME GO!

Will you hear me?

Yes, I believe you will. Because despite my faults, you care for me, not just as a citizen with rights but as a human being of dignity, I hope, and worth. What can possibly justify compulsary treatment when my *right to consent* implies, as well, my *right to refuse* treatment? You have always respected my wishes. You will respect them now, I trust, for they are no different from your own, so well expressed by the poet:

"Sustained and soothed
By an unfaltering trust, approach thy grave

Like one who wraps the drapery of his couch
About him, and lies down to pleasant dreams."**

### Rethink the Word "Euthanasia"

Crying "FOUL" and mindlessly labelling euthanasia a "dirty word," many Bible-thumping evangelists ignore situations such as faced by Augusta and by myriads of others who understand what we're saying. We're talking about the *sanctity of life,* not the preservation of a still-breathing corpse. Socrates is a classic example of one who preferred death to dishonor, extricating himself from degrading circumstances. Here we are talking of — not just euthanasia, but *Responsible Euthanasia.* To you who cringe at the word, remember. To many others, this word means peace, comfort, relief and literally, a good death.

I see my life, any life, as a candle, burning brightly. But in time when the wax dissolves, the wick wears down, may my wish be granted. As the candle flickers, let it go out. And let me fade, ever so gently, "into that good night."

---

**William Cullen Bryant, "Thanatopsis" A.D. 1811

## *EPILOGUE*
### *To Make Meaningful Their Days*

"Life is not breath but action,
the use of our senses, mind, faculties,
every part of ourselves which makes us
conscious of our being."
                Jean Jacques Rousseau

## *Epilogue*
## To Make Meaningful Their Days

Sign over the portal of a Midwestern bank:
*"Service is the rent we pay for the space we occupy in this world."*
"Nice thought," smiles the passing pedestrian. But what if he were an ailing octogenarian? "So I'm a drag. Seems I no longer deserve space in this world."

In subtle ways, America deflates her elders. Plagued by despair over what sociologists call their "roleless role," retired people commit more than 23% of all suicides, although they comprise 13% of the total population. What are they trying to tell us?

Cup your ears, America. Listen. Especially listen to the institutionalized who are saying: "Our few, precious, remaining years have no meaning — not to us, not to anybody. In this fast-paced world we're mothballed, irrelevant, rootless."

Grim, isn't it? Not that we say: "You're excess baggage." But from the look on our faces, the tone of our voices, they get the message. "Decent" people that we are, we can be heartless. To quote one nurse: "Cruelty can be so subtle that even the cruel don't recognize it."[1]

---

[1] Frances Storlie, R.N., *Nursing and the Social Conscience*, Appleton-Century-Crofts, N.Y.

This, so far is to set the stage. Before we can talk of helping elders to find meaning, we must see where and how we are failing to do so.

First of all, we delude ourselves. Flaunting that trendy word "holistic," we claim we are meeting the total needs of our elders. But are we?

In Chapter 9 the Maslow chart shows the five basic needs of any human being. Too many health care institutions focus primarily just on the first two — the body and safety needs. What about the other four, crucial to well being, imperative to mental health? (Needs for love, self-esteem, self-realization.) With exceptions, U.S. institutions come nowhere near meeting these total, life-affirming requirements. How can you tell? For one example, note the high incidence of depression among the long-lived.

"Come, come, Nancy," you may reply. "You're off base. You forget the spectacular strides the U.S. has made since the 1960s. Take those White House Conferences on Aging, from which sprang Senior Centers, Meals-on-Wheels and, in every state, Area Agencies on Aging. What about those myriads of new retirement-geriatric facilities — architectural marvels dotting the landscape? What about the Departments of Gerontology found today in most colleges and universities? Look at the barrage of books on aging! Note those national and international conferences on aging, the councils, the associations — all those free educational opportunities for the retired and all the special legislation enacted for their benefit as well as consumer advocate groups pushing for better nursing homes? We provide programs unmatched by any other nation. We deserve kudos. Well, don't we?"

**The Paradox**

Of course. And yet . . .

On the one hand we *can* be proud. These advances are great for the "young-old," those between ages 60 and 70. On the other hand we have not made the same progress for the "old-old." Despite public relations brochures which depict the nursing home as a "paradise-on-earth," there swirls a subtle undercurrent — that ceaseless lament among many residents: "What's there to get out of bed for each morning?"

"Nonsense, Nancy, you prophet of gloom and doom. Those

facilities all have super activities programs."

Alas, Friend, pitifully few residents actually get to go to activity sessions. There's no end of time on their hands. Many just sit and sit, staring at walls. If you need proof that life is meaningless for vast numbers of these people, I'll cite four examples.

## Example One:
## The Ongoing Problem of Abuse[2]

Although there *are* some "good" nursing homes (Chapter Six), which seek to put purpose in the lives of their clients, the problem of abuse runs rampant. So you thought abuse was snuffed out when, in the 1960s those scandals were exposed? So you believed that when the phrase "Nursing Home" was scrapped in favor of "Health Care Centers," the problems were licked? So you thought indignities ceased to exist when citizen action groups demanded reforms? Well, I have news for you. One cannot legislate caring. And although things look better today; although the worst abuses are found in a limited number of homes, very few facilities get off scott free. (Abuse runs rampant, too, in private residences.)

We need to define the word "abuse." As you know, abuse is not simply physical violence; not just slapping, whipping, forcing clients into sexual atrocities. Abuse can also mean bullying, shaming and verbal violence. Words devastate more than blows. Addressing a patient who had formerly practiced as a physician, an orderly shouted: "I don't care *who* you once were. Just you shut up because now and here you are nobody."

Isn't it abuse when all day a patient sits staring at walls, nothing to do, nobody to talk to? Isn't it abuse when for hours a male patient moans, begging to sit near his wife in the hall, but the aide quips: "Ha, ha — let him holler. Nobody tells *me* what to do!" And isn't it abuse, in fact horrendous violation of human rights when a woman, desperate for bladder relief, rings her call bell, yet nobody answers? So she puddles the floor. Whammo! *Now* she gets attention! She's shamed, humiliated, degraded. (By the way, our government blacklists *other nations* that violate human rights!)

---

[2]For further substantiation, see the December, 1984 issue of the "Journal of Geriatric Nursing." Slack, Inc. 6900 Grove Road, Thorofare, N.J. 08086

## Example Two:
### That Notorious "Rules and Regulations" Racket

In the U.S. we tie their hands, shackle their minds, stunt their initiative. I refer to that "rules and regulations" racket. Not permitted to make beds, set tables, water lawns, fix a shelf, distribute towels, dust knick-knacks? Why on earth not? (In the Soviet Union, for example, patients make eyeglass cases, and slippers for pay. Read in Chapter 10 how, in Chinese old age homes, they keep the geriatric patient busy and useful.) Forbidden, here, to make beds? Why? Because it's *against the rules!* Rules which are stupid, stifle the spirit. Rules conjured up for convenience of staff; rules which contribute nothing to client well being.

Just who invents these inhuman rules? Collectively it's inspectors, unions, health departments, bureaucrats, administrators, agencies, VIPs who have no background whatsoever in gerontology or psychology. That's who. It's people who are dead sure that "quality care" means simply: 1) Keep the premises neat and sanitary and 2) Adhere to fire and safety codes." "And yes," strut these "authorities," "if you don't we'll cite you for violations."

### Time to Cite for the Real Violations

Cite them, yes, by all means do so. But for heaven's sake, start citing for the *real* crimes, abuses that demean the human spirit. Time to cite and verbally flog that administrator who, when a client's relative makes a legitimate complaint, fires this cheap shot: "If you don't like it here you can always take your mother elsewhere!" Cite that aide with the instant solution: "Ignore him — he's senile!" Cite and throw to the wolves that nurse who cages her clients — denies them access to the out-of-doors. "No time," she says. No time for patients to hear the song of a robin, to inhale fresh air, to smell a flower, enjoy the color of a sunset? No time to revive their human spirits? (Do nurses deny themselves these privileges on days off?) And finally, cite and fire that employee who treats the elderly in rude and condescending ways. But first, boil all the above abusers in oil!

## Example Three
### That Perpetual "Short-of-Staff" Problem

Go visit your loved one in the hospital or nursing home, especially on a weekend or evening. A crisis arises. Try to find an aide. Ring the call bell. No response. Chase down the hall. Peek into every nook and cranny. Orderlies, aides, where are you? What's this, hide-and-seek?

Give up? Check the staff lounge. Ah, there they are, those few on duty, enjoying cokes, smokes, jokes. And why not? Except for the few with a strong sense of mission, why *should* they give a hoot for their jobs? Why should they bother with backrubs, or console a lonely patient? Here's why. *Low pay.* Minimum wage. Outrageous! What does this tell the employee? That he is not worth much: that his work is insignificant; that he need not respect his clients if they are not worth properly paid staff. Strange how staff works for crumbs, yet there is money for a new wing; money for a new facility; money for fancy equipment and decor!

Low pay invites staff turnover and staff shortages. Low pay equals low self-esteem. Low self-esteem produces sluggish caregiving. "You get what you pay for!"

The state of California finally got "schmart." They're providing 16 million dollars in additional reimbursements for increased wage levels.

### Example Four:
### The Disinterested Doctor

Many a doctor, scared of his/her own aging, sluffs off or avoids older patients like the Black Plague. In his clinic he quashes complaints with: "What do you expect, Gramps, it's your *age.* Nothing I can do!"

The next time you hear such unprofessional bosh, string that doctor up from the highest branch. He's afflicted with "ageism," that malady which slams the door on treatment for countless legitimate candidates. He sits behind his desk, blissfully unaware that geriatrics, rather than just keeping organisms alive, is the art of maintaining vigorous people. He doesn't know that our elders, far from being "waste products of society" (a term I've actually heard used), are one of our nation's great assets in terms of wisdom, experience and links to our heritage. He hasn't heard that they, too, are human beings.

Why such ignorance? Hear this. Most medical schools fail to teach geriatrics and gerontology. Check the curriculum directory of the latest AAMC publication* and note that, as of this printing, only 20 of our 126 medical schools list geriatrics as a course.

*American Association of Medical Colleges

The remainder claim that they integrate the subject (or should we say "dilute") into basic science courses. In the U.S., geriatrics is not a specialty as it is in Canada and the United Kingdom. In fact in Scotland, you cannot graduate without geriatrics from the University of Edinburgh. In only ten schools is a gerontology course listed!

As U.S. physicians debate whether or not to make geriatrics, like pediatrics, a specialty, it seems that, until they do — (and there are complicated pros and cons, say the doctors) physicians will continue to misunderstand the aging process and how it affects mind and body. They'll keep right on misdiagnosing, under or overtreating, prescribing the tranquilizer as a panacea for everything from hangnails to halitosis. And many elders will continue to waste away to a tragic, doddering end.

We do salute, however, those physicians (whose numbers are growing) who practice preventive and holistic medicine — those who abhor age discrimination; those who see the vast potential of creative geriatric medicine. This next message is not for them.

### Memo to the Medical Profession

"Tempus fugit." Soon *you'll* be joining the "Grand Generation" and then, tell me, will you be content to grovel for the same scrawny scraps you now toss to your older clients? When will you scrap that de-da de-da de-da de-da broken record on which your voice keeps playing: "Just keep him comfortable — nothing I can do!"

Hold it, Doctor. There's *plenty* you can do. Replacing the cobwebs that clutter your mind, you can review the research findings of our great gerontology centers such as UCLA, Johns Hopkins, Duke and Miami U and discover that:

1) Memory loss is not a natural function of age
2) Sexuality has no age limits
3) Intelligence does not necessariy decline with age
4) Rather than age itself, it is cultural and emotional factors which most frequently induce chronic brain syndrome.

And something else you can do. In treating elders, when did you last take into consideration the heavy stresses, the cumulative losses through death and separation, the anxiety engendered by financial and physical setbacks? Way back then, even Socrates knew that "without cure of the emotions, there is no cure of the body."

But the best thing you can do is to quit footdragging and start leading. You know that the older generation is the fastest growing segment in our society. Then why are you not more aggressive in wiping out those myths which run rampant in the very institutions where you practice? You could be changing societal attitudes, teaching prevention, curing, or reversing many physical and mental ills. Myths such as:

*Most aged are ill and disabled.*
*Most suffer from mental deterioration.*
*"Senility" is incurable and irreversible.*
*Older people have no sexual interest or activity.*
*Drug therapy for the aged is the same as for anyone else.*
*You can't teach an old dog new tricks.*
*Old people have worked hard all their lives:*
  *they need their rest.*
*Reminiscing is boring - you shouldn't allow it.*
*Most families just "dump" their relative in a home*
  *because they don't really care.*
*If you live long enough, you'll become sick,*
  *senile, sexless and senseless!*

You've made a start — I'll grant you that. On the horizon looms the "teaching nursing home," affiliated with a center of learning. A few geriatric fellowships are on the road.

But hurry! You'd jolly well better jump on the bandwagon or else the American public, ever less patient, will have you jumping on hot coals!

Now to the crux of this chapter. So far we've seen what is not being done; how sticky issues in health care stem mostly from poor attitudes, low expectation. Using your creative powers, you professionals, paraprofessionals and lay persons can offer antidotes. You can't *make* patients happy. But you *can* facilitate the environment. You can help enormously to open up the paths and to:

## Make Meaningful Their Days

Try this. *Latch on to Life Roles.* That's what they did with my father. Paralyzed, aphasic, depressed, he entered the nursing home at age 78. But things picked up. His speech returned, his life regained meaning. And, amazingly, until he died at age 95, he remained motivated. (How often does this happen in an institution?) What miracle took place?

No magic. Just a simple approach which can be applied to any patient, young, old, ambulatory or bedridden. Staff became excited over the idea of latching on to life roles. But the impact didn't hit me until I saw what it did for my Dad.

One day, visiting Father, I blew my top. "Good Heavens, Father," I cried. "Look at you! Today it's beans on your vest. Last week it was egg on your chin. Enough! I'm hauling you out of here. I'm putting you in a home where you'll get more meticulous care!"

"Oh no you don't," yelled Father, almost plunging from his wheelchair. "I won't hear of it. Who would counsel the lonely? Who would assist at Sunday and weekday services?"

Father had been a minister. And staff, bless their brains, used this knowledge to keep his spark alive. They let him do what he used to do, what he liked to do, what he did best. With a sense of control over his life, Father was still "somebody."

I ate my words. Rather than subject him to a traumatic transfer, I first made sure that staff rectified that "egg-on-chin" problem. Next I encouraged him to retain his sense of mission. Tremendous, the way he was "paying rent for the space he occupied!"

Most patients once had a job, career, avocation which put a spark in their eyes. Wherever possible, *resurrect this interest.* Even if only partially. Look over there at old Mrs. Hansen — wasn't she once famous around the block for her "sticky buns?" How can her expertise be utilized here? Has she chatted with the dietician? And what about Mr. Stein, landscape designer, or that young patient John Denton? Could their knowledge contribute somehow to the needs of the facility? Be creative. Don't slam the door on them with "No way," or "No time." Enlist volunteers to carry on the process. Open the paths because, as psychologist John Valusek bluntly states: *"It is immoral to interfere with the potential of others."*

George is a young student paralyzed from the neck down. But his caregivers latched on to his obsession with mathematics. At first, hopelessly depressed, today George is learning computer science, tutoring a child and working towards his Masters degree. It gives me gooseflesh — the potential in almost anybody! You've read of Elizabeth, also with quadraplegic problems, who wants to die, begs to go. So would I with no reason to live. Before it's too late, latch on to her life role, put the spotlight on her abilities, rather than her disabilities. There is no such word as "hopeless" unless it applies to staff or family attitudes.

*One Word of Caution:* Lest we fall into the trap of viewing activities, per se, as the only satisfactions, keep in mind those who voluntarily refrain from planned programs; those who derive meaning from meditation and aloneness. Declared one such woman: "Potholders are not for everyone!" Neither depressed nor copping out, this person draws meaning and contentment from her own inner resources. Be on the lookout for her kind.

So your clients are kept clean and neat? So staff and family are kind to them? That's enough? That's *all* they need? Hold it! Hear that commotion up there? Why it's Father, pounding his cane on Heaven's floor. "Hey you folks down there," he's shouting. "That's not the half of it!"

We hear you, Pa. You remind us that life for the young or old means more than pills, pulses and prostheses. It means that we:

. . . know who the person was and what he could do;

. . . know who the person is and what he now can do;

. . . know who the person may become and what he may yet achieve.

Far from being a "drag," our handicapped of all ages can and many do earn their space in this world. For most of them, living longer can mean living better *if we pave the way.* Life is for the living. For the rest of their time, their one and only sojourn on this earth, we must seize the challenge, repay them for the beauty they have brought into our lives.

We will help to *make their days meaningful.*

**FINAL CURTAIN**

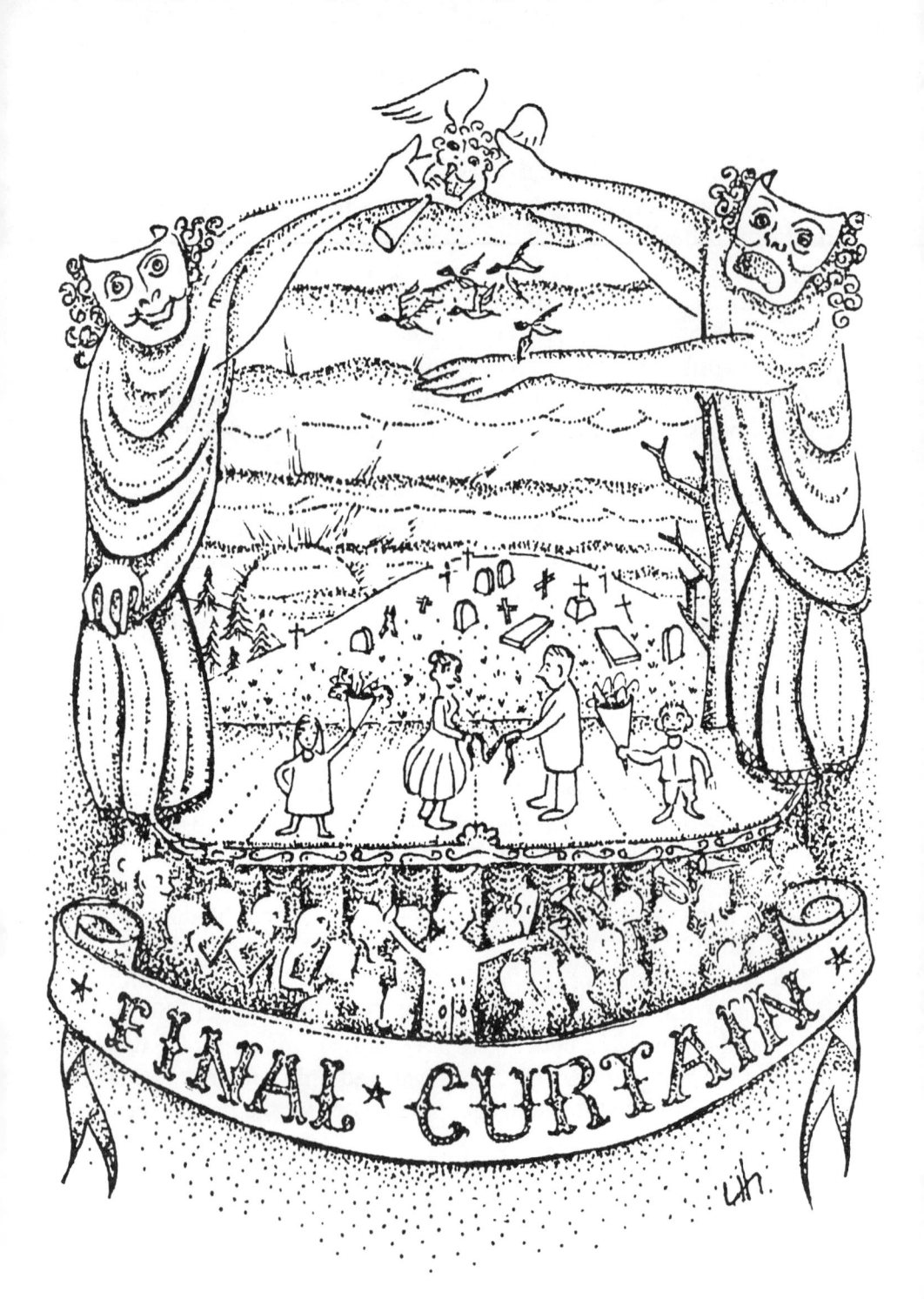

# TO THE READER, A CONCLUDING WORD OF MOTIVATION

Yes, in today's health care field, we are confronted with many "sticky issues." Each of us, if we care enough, if we speak out, will come UNDER CROSSFIRE from those with vested interests, those who are power-hungry, those who have lost sight of the patient as a person.

My challenge to you? Keep up the barrage. Speak out. For, as Charles Mackay wrote before the turn of the century:

> YOU HAVE NO ENEMIES, YOU SAY?
> ALAS, MY FRIEND, THE BOAST IS POOR -
>
> HE WHO HAS MINGLED IN THE FRAY
> OF DUTY, THAT THE BRAVE ENDURE,
> MUST HAVE MADE FOES! IF YOU HAVE NONE,
> SMALL IS THE WORK THAT YOU HAVE DONE.
>
> YOU'VE HIT NO TRAITOR ON THE HIP,
> YOU'VE DASHED NO CUP FROM PERJURED LIP,
> YOU'VE NEVER TURNED THE WRONG TO RIGHT,
> YOU'VE BEEN A COWARD IN THE FIGHT!

With all the social conscience; with all the caring individuals and dedicated organizations which abound in our land, we can ward off that crossfire. We can embrace the marvelous philosophy of that public-spirited person who said:

> "I'd rather live fifty years as a lion
> than one hundred years as a chicken!"

- *The End* -